Movement Sciences: Transfer of Knowledge into Pediatric Therapy Practice

Movement Sciences: Transfer of Knowledge into Pediatric Therapy Practice has been co-published simultaneously as *Physical & Occupational Therapy in Pediatrics*, Volume 24, Numbers 1/2 2004.

Movement Sciences: Transfer of Knowledge into Pediatric Therapy Practice

Robert J. Palisano, PT, ScD
Editor

Movement Sciences: Transfer of Knowledge into Pediatric Therapy Practice has been co-published simultaneously as *Physical & Occupational Therapy in Pediatrics*, Volume 24, Numbers 1/2 2004.

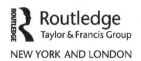

Routledge
Taylor & Francis Group

NEW YORK AND LONDON

First Published by

The Haworth Press, Inc., 10 Alice Street, Binghamton, NY 13904-11580 USA

Transferred to Digital Printing 2009 by Routledge
711 Third Ave, New York NY 10017
2 Park Square, Milton Park, Abingdon, Oxon, OX14 4RN

Movement Sciences: Transfer of Knowledge into Pediatric Therapy Practice has been co-published simultaneously as *Physical & Occupational Therapy in Pediatrics*™, Volume 24, Numbers 1/2 2004.

The development, preparation, and publication of this work has been undertaken with great care. However, the publisher, employees, editors, and agents of The Haworth Press and all imprints of The Haworth Press, Inc., including The Haworth Medical Press® and Pharmaceutical Products Press®, are not responsible for any errors contained herein or for consequences that may ensue from use of materials or information contained in this work. Opinions expressed by the author(s) are not necessarily those of The Haworth Press, Inc. With regard to case studies, identities and circumstances of individuals discussed herein have been changed to protect confidentiality. Any resemblance to actual persons, living or dead, is entirely coincidental.

Cover design by Lora Wiggins

Library of Congress Cataloging-in-Publication Data

Movement sciences : transfer of knowledge into pediatric therapy practice / Robert J. Palisano, editor.
     p. ; cm.
     "Co-published simultaneously as Physical & occupational therapy in pediatrics, volume 24, numbers 1/2 2004."
     Includes bibliographical references and index.
     ISBN 0-7890-2560-4 (hard cover : alk. paper) – ISBN 0-7890-2561-2 (soft cover : alk. paper)
     1. Physical therapy for children. 2. Occupational therapy for children. 3. Motor learning. 4. Motor ability in children. 5. Cerebral palsied children. [DNLM: 1. Movement–physiology–Child. 2. Physical Therapy Techniques–Child. WB 460 M935 2004] I. Palisano, Robert J.
RJ53.P5M68 2004
615.8'2'083–dc22
                                          2004008133

Movement Sciences: Transfer of Knowledge into Pediatric Therapy Practice

CONTENTS

INTRODUCTION

Movement science provides foundation knowledge for pediatric physical therapy and occupational therapy practice. Movement science is a multidisciplinary field of study that includes motor control, motor learning, motor development, biomechanics, cognitive psychology, and ecology. A common focus is the understanding of human movement behavior. Knowledge of motor control, learning and development of children with movement disorders informs pediatric therapy practice. Topics addressed in this special volume include: motor control of posture and prehension, motor learning challenges, predictors of standing balance, the effect of environment setting on mobility, and measurement of muscle extensibility in newborns.

On a daily basis, pediatric physical therapists and occupational therapists are challenged to apply knowledge of movement science to clinical practice. To what extent does this occur? In health care, current research often is not applied or transfer into practice is slow (Chassin & Galvin, 1998). Perhaps research is a necessary but not a sufficient condition for application of knowledge into practice. Haynes, Devereau and Guyatt (2002) state that "evidence alone does not make decisions, people do." Therapists must apply movement science research in ways that address the needs of children and families. Interventions must be acceptable to children and families and meaningful to their daily life. Therapist perspective, child and family preference, and environmental

[Haworth co-indexing entry note]: "Introduction" Palisano, Robert J. Co-published simultaneously in *Physical & Occupational Therapy in Pediatrics* (The Haworth Press, Inc.) Vol. 24, No. 1/2, 2004, pp. 1-3; and: *Movement Sciences: Transfer of Knowledge into Pediatric Therapy Practice* (ed: Robert J. Palisano) The Haworth Press, Inc., 2004, pp. 1-3. Single or multiple copies of this article are available for a fee from The Haworth Document Delivery Service [1-800-HAWORTH, 9:00 a.m. - 5:00 p.m. (EST). E-mail address: docdelivery@haworthpress.com].

Digital Object Identifier: 10.1300/J006v24n01_01

context are factors that likely influence how knowledge is transferred into practice.

The focus of this publication is on transfer of knowledge of movement science into pediatric physical and occupational therapy practice. Winstein and Knecht (1990) state that knowledge of movement science is often not directly translatable to practice. They advocate that therapists should be consumers of knowledge and capable of determining how research is best applied to practice. The authors of this special volume are both competent researchers and experienced practitioners. As scientist-practitioners, they are able to analyze interventions in light of current knowledge. Their ability to "think outside the box" when considering the implications of their research and "fill gaps" in knowledge with frameworks for decision-making exemplifies knowledge transfer.

The articles reflect the author's expertise and include models for practice and original research reports:

- *Sarah Westcott* and *Pat Burtner* analyze research on postural control in children from the perspectives of systems theory, reactive, and anticipatory control. They present suggestions for an evidence-based approach to improving postural control at the impairment and functional activity levels.
- *Linda Pax Lowes, Sarah Westcott, Bob Palisano, Susan Effgen,* and *Margo Orlin* present research that indicates that muscle force production and joint range of motion are highly related to standing balance in children with spastic cerebral palsy. Implications are presented for exercise, task specific strengthening and range of motion, community-based recreation, and use of orthotics.
- *Joanne Valvano* presents her model for activity-based interventions for children with neurological disorders. This article provides a conceptual framework for adapting motor learning strategies to meet the needs of children with neuromuscular impairments.
- *Beth Tieman, Bob Palisano, Ed Gracely, Peter Rosenbaum, Lisa Chiarello,* and *Maggie O'Neil* report that mobility methods of children with cerebral palsy change in a non-linear pattern over time and across home, school, and outdoor/community settings. Potential changes in the child, the environment, and in person-environment interaction are discussed and recommendations are provided for examination and evaluation.
- *Sue Duff* and *Jeanne Charles* review the development of prehension in infants and children from a motor control perspective. The authors apply a framework for development of motor control that in-

cludes adaptability, anticipatory control, unimanual and bimanual coordination, and object manipulation.

• *Marybeth Grant-Beuttler, Peter Leininger,* and *Bob Palisano* suggest that determining the influence of muscle and tendon length on active muscle force production has implications for understanding preterm motor development and decisions regarding the need for early intervention. They present evidence that a measure of extensibility of the gastrocnemius-soleus muscle is reliable in fullterm and preterm newborns.

When reading this special volume, you are encouraged to reflect on your practice. How do the authors' perspectives and research findings apply to the children and families on your caseload? How do their frameworks for intervention compare with your preferred intervention strategies and procedures? Hopefully you will discuss the articles with colleagues and provide the authors feedback, either directly or in a letter to the editor. Most important, reflect on the articles when providing services to children and families. In doing so, you will become an active participant in transfer of knowledge of movement science into pediatric physical therapy and occupational therapy practice.

Robert J. Palisano, PT, ScD
Drexel University

REFERENCES

Chassin, M. R., & Galvin, R. W. (1998). The urgent need to improve health care quality: Institute of Medicine National Roundtable on Health Care Quality. *Journal of the American Medical Association, 280*: 1000-1005.

Haynes, R. B., Devereau, P. J., & Guyatt, G. H. (2002). Physicians' and patient choices in evidence based practice. *British Medical Journal, 324*: 1350.

Winstein, C. J., & Knecht, H. G. (1990). Movement science and its relevance to physical therapy. *Physical Therapy, 70*: 759-762.

Postural Control in Children:
Implications for Pediatric Practice

Sarah L. Westcott
Patricia Burtner

SUMMARY. Based on a systems theory of motor control, reactive postural control (RPA) and anticipatory postural control (APA) in children are reviewed from several perspectives in order to develop an evidence-based intervention strategy for improving postural control in children with limitations in motor function. Research on development of postural control, postural control in children with specific motor disabilities, and interventions to improve postural control is analyzed. A strategy for intervention to improve postural control systems at the impairment and functional activity levels based on a systems theoretical perspective is presented. Suggestions for research to improve evidence for best practice are provided. *[Article copies available for a fee from The Haworth Document Delivery Service: 1-800-HAWORTH. E-mail address: <docdelivery@ haworthpress.com> Website: <http://www.HaworthPress.com> © 2004 by The Haworth Press, Inc. All rights reserved.]*

Sarah L. Westcott is Adjunct Associate Professor at Drexel University, Programs in Rehabilitation Sciences, Philadelphia, PA, and a staff physical therapist at the Lake Washington School District, Redmond, WA, and Northwest Pediatric Therapies, Issaquah, WA. Patricia Burtner is Associate Professor at University of New Mexico, Occupational Therapy Programs, Albuquerque, NM.

Address correspondence to: Sarah L. Westcott, PT, PhD, 5019 218th Avenue NE, Redmond, WA 98053 (E-mail: wests@isomedia.com).

[Haworth co-indexing entry note]: "Postural Control in Children: Implications for Pediatric Practice." Westcott, Sarah L., and Patricia Burtner. Co-published simultaneously in *Physical & Occupational Therapy in Pediatrics* (The Haworth Press, Inc.) Vol. 24, No. 1/2, 2004, pp. 5-55; and: *Movement Sciences: Transfer of Knowledge into Pediatric Therapy Practice* (ed: Robert J. Palisano) The Haworth Press, Inc., 2004, pp. 5-55. Single or multiple copies of this article are available for a fee from The Haworth Document Delivery Service [1-800-HAWORTH, 9:00 a.m. - 5:00 p.m. (EST). E-mail address: docdelivery@haworthpress.com].

Digital Object Identifier: 10.1300/J006v24n01_02

KEYWORDS. Reactive postural adjustments, anticipatory postural adjustments, children, physical therapy, occupational therapy

INTRODUCTION

Movement is a core feature of our being human. Through movement, we care for ourselves and express our feelings and desires. We generally perform movements with ease and dexterity, yet the act of moving is incredibly complex and somewhat vulnerable as evidenced by the existence of movement disorders. Due to the complexity of movement generation and in an effort to understand the etiology of movement disorders, we have sought to find ways to break down the act of moving into components that we can measure, analyze, and apply to intervention. For instance, movement can be broken down into the components for generating and executing the "primary" or desired movement and the components for the background postural movement necessary to support that prime movement (Massion, 1992). Massion (1992) compares a motor act to an iceberg, with the goal oriented movement being the apparent ice and the postural related component of the movement being the hidden ice. Controversy exists as to whether postural and prime movements should be considered separately, however, recent studies have supported the existence of separate neural control mechanisms for postural and primary movements (Aruin, Shiratori, & Latash, 2001; Slijper, Latash, & Mordkoff, 2002). Postural movement has also been demonstrated to be a basic ability and critical link for producing coordinated movement (Katic, Bonacin, & Blazevic, 2001) and one that is lacking in many pediatric movement disorders (Westcott, 2001). Tests and measures have been created to examine postural control (Westcott, Richardson, & Lowes, 1997) and many prominent intervention methods emphasize the facilitation of postural control (Westcott, 2001).

Postural control for movement involves the orientation of the body in space for stability as well as orientation to the task within the context of the environment (Massion, 1994). At times the body is controlled at rest (static equilibrium) and other times with movement (dynamic equilibrium). Postural control can be defined simply as the ability to control one's center of mass (COM) over the base of support (BOS) (Horak, 1992). It can be broken down into several units as depicted in Figure 1. These units hypothetically vary in their safety vs. efficiency effect as characterized in Figure 1. Two of these units will be considered in detail in this paper, the control mechanisms for reacting to unexpected external postural perturbations, *reactive postural adjustments* (RPA), and

FIGURE 1. Components of postural strategies presented along a time and efficiency scale. Earlier postural preparations are safer but not as efficient in terms of producing coordinated movements. Anticipatory postural adjustments, occurring within 100 msec of the prime movement onset, are more efficient than postural preparations and assist in the coordination and safety of the prime movement activity. Reactive postural adjustments occur after the prime movement or in reaction to external perturbations, within 80-100 msec, and are very efficient in facilitating postural control. (Adapted from Frank & Earl, 1990; Liu, 2001)

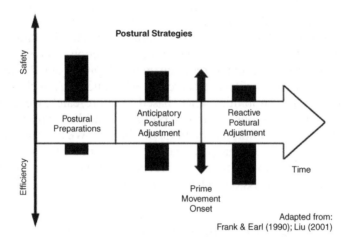

those for anticipating internal postural perturbations related to production of voluntary movement, *anticipatory postural adjustments* (APA). An example of a RPA is the response that occurs to keep the body balanced when someone bumps into you. An APA example is the postural activity that precedes and links with a reach forward while standing so that you do not lose your balance and the movement is completed smoothly and accurately.

Applying a general systems theory of motor control, within both RPA and APA, there are several systems that coordinate to produce effective postural control (Bernstein, 1967; Horak, 1992). At least three systems, *sensory*, *motor*, and *musculoskeletal*, participate in coordinating postural activity. The sensory system cues the individual that there has been a perturbation and/or gives feedback for adjustments during slow movements and after movements in regard to how successful the postural activity generated has been. The motor system organizes and cues the appropriate activation of the muscles. The musculoskeletal system provides the framework on which we move and creates the forces to produce the postural muscle activity. The state of any of these systems affects the overall postural activity and in a sense may control the output. Other systems can also have an effect on the postural activity observed. For instance, the directions given to the individual, or the behavioral state and alertness of the individual may vary the postural activity (Burleigh & Horak, 1996; Burleigh, Horak, & Malouin, 1994; Nashner, 1982). Likewise the environment and task can cause the individual to vary postural activity (Thelan & Spencer, 1998). Figure 2, which depicts postural control from a systems theory perspective, provides the conceptual framework for this article.

The purpose of this paper is to summarize research on postural control (RPA and APA) in children and to present intervention strategies based on our summary. First, we review research on development of RPA and APA. Next we analyze the available research on RPA and APA in children with and without motor disabilities. Then, based on our research, we discuss the evidence for interventions to improve postural control and present an intervention strategy for children with motor disabilities. We have taken the liberty to make suggestions that potentially follow from the research, but also may overstep the specific research evidence. We have done this deliberately to generate discussion and encourage further research.

DEVELOPMENT OF RPA AND APA

Incorporating research from the fields of neuroscience and biomechanics, our understanding of the development of postural control is based on the development of neural and musculoskeletal systems. Three processes critical to underlying postural mechanisms have been identified as: (1) *motor processes*: the emergence of neuromuscular response synergies which maintain stability of the neck, trunk and legs, (2) *sensory processes*: the development of visual, vestibular and somatosensory systems, as well as the maturation of central sensory strategies organizing outputs from these senses for body and limb orientation, and (3) *musculoskeletal components*: changes in structural and soft tissue morphology, muscle strength development, and range of motion which includes the biomechanical linkage of body segments for movement (Shumway-Cook & Woollacott, 2001). These systems develop in a non-linear fashion at different rates. Postural control in the child emerges when development of each system reaches the threshold necessary to support the specific motor behavior (Thelan, 1986).

FIGURE 2. Postural control components based on a systems theory of motor control. The task, environment and child represent systems affecting movement. Within the child, the movement system can be divided into the control components for the prime movement and postural control. Within postural control, the sensory, motor and musculoskeletal systems work in concert with other systems to produce efficient and safe postures and recovery of postures. These three systems have been examined to some extent in children with and without disabilities. (Adapted from Horak, 1991; Liu, 2001)

Postural Control Systems Theory

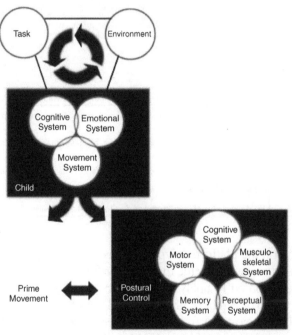

Thus, knowledge of the development of each system is important for determining which system may be *rate limiting*. Through identification of the system(s) that are rate limiting, the therapist is able to formulate an intervention plan specific to the needs of the individual child. Table 1 A-D details the developmental progression for each system for RPA and APA.

In the research summarized in Table 1, a common paradigm used to determine the RPA is to place the child on a moveable platform and translate the platform in anterior or posterior directions to produce external perturbations (Nashner, 1976) (see Figure 3). The child can be supine, prone, sitting

TABLE 1A. Typical Development of Postural Control: Musculoskeletal System (Mattiello & Woollacott, 1997; Shumway-Cook & Woollacott, 2001; Woollacott & Shumway-Cook, 1994)

Components	Age of maturation to adult-like capacity
Force production (Breniere & Bril, 1998; Lin, Brown, & Walsh, 1994; Roncesvalles & Jensen, 1993; Roncesvalles, Woollacott, & Jensen, 2001; Schloon, O'Brien, Scholten & Prechtl, 1976; Sundermier, Woollacott, Roncesvalles & Jensen, 2001)	2 months–force generation against gravity in neck muscles when tilted in prone and supine 6 months (pre-pull-to-stand infants)–force generation adequate to sustain body weight Under 1 year age–low force production capability is a constraint for sitting and standing 9 months-10 years (developing through life)–overall torque production to recover balance after sudden perturbation increases; peak torque at the ankle and hip increased as distance and time to complete COP readjustments decreased; newly standing and walking infants have smaller torque values than older children who are able to skip and gallop Postural capacity to control balance with leg muscles may not be complete until *4-5 years of walking experience*
Range of Motion	Developing through the teen years; Should not be a constraint until elderly
Body Geometry (Jensen & Bothner, in press; McCollum & Leen, 1989; Woollacott, Roseblad, & von Hofsten, 1988)	Different ages–changes rapidly during growth spurts dependent on gender and hormonal development Infants–increased body mass in head, arms, and trunk segments as compared to older children and adults 12-15 months–increased upper body mass results in faster sway during perturbed stance 4-9 years–kinematics of body sway similar to adults 12-15 years through adults–gradual decrease in sway velocities

or standing on the platform. Typically electromyographic (EMG) recordings are used to determine the muscle coordination patterns used and kinematics are recorded to analyze specific body movements. The center of pressure (COP) or center of gravity (COG) position changes of an individual can also be recorded from force plates to document RPA during any type of external perturbation or APA during any type of voluntary movement (Liu, 2001) (see Figure 4). RPA changes due to sensory input differences have been examined using a sensory organization test consisting of six conditions which systematically alter the visual and somatosensory input to determine if a person over-relies on or has decreased registration of a particular sensory input to maintain balance (Horak, Shumway-Cook, & Black, 1988) (see Figure 5). Readers are encouraged to refer to the studies referenced throughout this paper to fully understand the methods.

To summarize, for RPA, there appear to be innate patterns of muscle coordination organized for head control, sitting balance and standing bal-

TABLE 1B. Typical Development of Postural Control: Sensory System (Forssberg & Nashner, 1982; Hirschfeld & Forssberg, 1994; Shumway-Cook & Woollacott, 1985a; Westcott, Zaino, Miller, & Thorpe, 1997; Woollacott, Shumway-Cook & Williams, 1989; Woollacott et al., 1998)

Components	Age of maturation to adult-like capacity
Vision (Foster, Sviestrup, & Woollacott, 1996; Jouen, 1984, 1988,1993, in press; Lee & Aronson, 1974; Sundermier & Woollacott, 1998; Woollacott, Debu, & Mowatt, 1987)	Birth–sensory receptor mature; 3-4-day-old infants show activation of neck muscles to visual flow patterns; acuity improves for distance vision over first year 2 months–preference for reliance on visual input for head control Birth to 1 year–visual preference for postural orientation corrections for sitting balance 13-16 months–visual preference for independent standing to early walking 2-10 years (experienced walkers)–show decreased sway magnitude and falls during standing balance challenges from a "moving room" visual input Birth to death–vision used as primary information when first learning a task or in a novel environment
Somatosensory (cutaneous and proprioceptive) (Lee & Aronson, 1974)	Birth–sensory receptor mature 6 months or greater–can use somatosensory inputs for head compensatory responses and maintenance of sitting balance 4-6 years–show beginning ability to use somatosensory input for sensory conflict resolution 7-10 years–show adult-like ability to use somatosensory input for sensory conflict resolution
Vestibular (Cherng, Chen, & Su, 2001; Jouen, 1984, 1988,1993, in press)	Birth–sensory receptor mature 7-10 years–can use vestibular input as the reference system in a near adult-like manner for resolution of sensory conflict, but sway area and amplitude are greater than young adults (19-23 years).
Sensory conflict resolution / Sensory integration	4-6 years–higher sway & greater variability in sensory conflict conditions 7-10 years–can choose and select sensory information accurately for maintenance of postural control

ance. There also appear to be periods in development where infants and children become more disorganized and regress to immature muscle co-contraction patterns to potentially reduce the degrees of freedom they need to control. With experience and practice, these co-contractions decrease, allowing more flexible and adaptable RPA. There appears to be a stage-like RPA development with disorganization in standing postural motor coordination patterns at 4-6 years age, possibly due to growth spurts or development of the sensory organization necessary for postural control. Sensory system organization for postural control proceeds from the individual being visually dependent for maintenance of balance to the ability to maintain balance based upon subtle somatosensory inputs.

TABLE 1C. Typical Development of Postural Control: Motor System–RPA (Shumway-Cook & Woollacott, 1985; Woollacott, Shumway-Cook & Williams, 1989; Woollacott et al., 1998)

Motor skill	Age of maturation to adult-like capacity
Head Stabilization: (Schloon, O'Brien, & Scholten, 1976; Prechtl & Hopkins, 1986)	0-7 weeks (pre-antigravity head control)–Active muscle bursts during active head turning 8-10 week–clear EMG patterns of neck musculature 2-months–head control complete
Sitting: (Muscle Coordination Patterns [MCPs]) (Hadders-Algra et al., 1996, 1998a, 1998b; Hirschfeld & Forssberg, 1994; Shepherd, 1995)	3-5 months (pre-sitting infant)–Practice of antigravity extensor and flexor muscles in prone & supine; single postural muscle groups activated or antagonist activated rather than an identifiable sequence 5-6 months (able to sit with arm support)–Activation of directionally specific MCPs (agonists opposite to the side the child is falling) but slow & variable timing (co-contractions & reversals of proximal to distal patterns) & poor adaptation to task specific conditions 7-10 months (sitting infant)–decreased timing variability of directionally specific MCPs (activations of leg, trunk, neck muscles) 9 months-3 years (transient toddling phase)–invariant use of directionally specific MCPs, some use of co-contractions; good modulation of pelvic muscles at BOS for adaptations to task specific conditions ~3 years to adulthood–variability in directionally specific MCPs, less co-contraction & use of neck muscles to improve variability of postural control
Standing: (Forssberg & Nashner, 1982; Hadders-Algra et al., 1998; Roncesvalles, Woollacott, & Jensen, 2000; Sveistrup et al., 1990; Woollacott, & Sveistrup, 1992; Sveistrup & Woollacott, 1996)	2-6 months (pre-sitting infants)–no identifiable muscle organization noted 7-8 months (infants who pull-to-stand)–show beginnings of ankle strategies 10-12 months (independent standers)–adult-like RPA with grossly directionally specific (distal to proximal) MCPs 12-16 months (toddlers)–More consistent directionally specific MCPs although onset latencies longer With ~ 3 months walking experience, compensatory stepping balance responses emerge. ~4-6 years–Variability of MCPs occurs (perhaps due to growth spurts or sensory integration changes) 7-10 years–Adult-like use of directionally specific MCPs Other determinants of RPA MCP choice: type of surface standing on; availability of sensory cues; instructions for task, regularity for perturbations.

However, at transition stages (e.g., beginning to sit, beginning to stand), visual dependence re-emerges until the child gains more stability. The ability to resolve sensory conflicts matures gradually to an adult-like state at 7-10 years of age. Development of APA seems to follow a similar sequence as RPA, however, the patterns of motor coordination are more

TABLE 1D. Typical Development of Postural Control: Motor System–APA (Shumway-Cook & Woollacott, 1985; Woollacott, Shumway-Cook & Williams, 1989; Woollacott et al., 1998)

Motor skill	Age of maturation to adult-like capacity
Movement in sitting:	4 months–complex APA in sitting, but infrequent
(Van der Fits & Hadders-Algra, 1998; Van der Fits, Klip, van Eykern, & Hadders-Algra, 1999; Van der Fits, Otten, Klip, Van Eykern, & Hadders-Algra, 1999)	6-8 months–less APA than at 4 months in sitting; at 8 months more ample APA and can adapt to different sitting positions and velocities of prime movement 12-15 months–consistent APA, particularly in neck muscles
Movement in standing:	
(Assaiante, Woollacott, & Amblard, 2000; Berger, Quintern, & Deitz, 1985; Forssberg & Nashner, 1982 Hass, Diener, Rapp & Dichgans, 1989; Hay & Redon, 1999, 2001; Hirschfeld & Forssberg, 1991, 1992; Riach & Hayes, 1990; Schmitz, Martin, & Assaiante, 1999; Westcott & Zaino, 1997; Witherington, von Hofsten, Rosander et al., 2002; Woollacott & Jensen, 1996)	10-13 months–occasional APA 16-17 months–more consistent and temporally specific APA; ability to modulate APA related to experience with activity and time that stood independently & walked alone 3-4 years–variable APA in a load release task 4-6 years–APAs recorded in the following tasks: lever pull; voluntary drop weight; tip-toe stand; raise arm. APA may shift from a supporting function to movement to a compensatory function of postural stability. 6-8 years–variable APAs in stand and reach task 9-12 years–more consistent APAs in stand and reach; less APA activity, i.e., more tolerant to unbalanced situation; modulation of APA in weighted and un-weighted wrist reach task. All ages–APA dependent on task; mature after RPA in a posture and after experience with movement in the posture. First APA response in a new movement is a co-contraction (freezing the degrees of freedom), then after practice, more variability in APA and movement occurs (Vereiiken et al., 1992).
Movement during gait initiation (GI)	Infants learning to walk– can apply necessary force to contact surface in anticipation of body sway
(Assaiante, 1998; Assaiante et al., 2000; Breniere & Bril, 1998; Ledebt, Bril, & Breniere, 1998; Malouin & Richards, 2000	2.5 years–GI APA present; young walkers *(1-17 months walking experience)* use lateral shifts of COP (rather than adult-like posterior shifts) & use upper and lower body to make the shifts; begin to show lower activation of proximal muscle groups & higher activation of ankle muscles 4-6 years–GI APA demonstrate adult-like patterns of EMG and COP; with *4-5 years walking experience*, postural control MCPs move distally with ability to control gravitational forces with leg muscles during gait 6-8 years–GI APA coordinated with the velocity of the step forward as in adults

variable and appear to depend more on practice and learning through experience, resulting in APA appropriate for specific tasks and environments. Fortunately for therapists, both nature and nurture seem to be involved with the development and variations of learning postural control (Hadders-Algra, Brogen, & Forssberg, 1997).

FIGURE 3. Moving platform with horizontal translations in anterior-posterior plane resulting in perturbation of children's balance in (a) sitting and (b) standing. Reactive postural adjustments are identified through electromyography of postural muscles and force measures in platform (Adapted from Shumway-Cook & Woollacott, 2001)

A. Sitting protocol

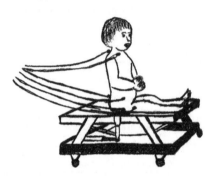

B. Standing protocol

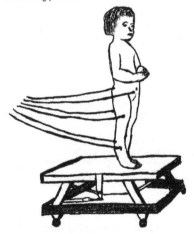

FIGURE 4. An example of anticipatory postural adjustments (APA) center of pressure (COP) movement during a stand and reach activity. Time is represented along the x-axis and the mm of movement of the COP in the anterior (up) and posterior (down) direction. The top figure represents a child with spastic diplegia, GMFCS level II, who had had a selective dorsal rhizotomy. The bottom figure is an age matched child with typical development. The reach movement onset is represented by the dashed line and both graphs are aligned by the reach movement. The child with CP shows later onset of the posterior shift of the APA COP and less amplitude (Adapted from Liu, 2001)

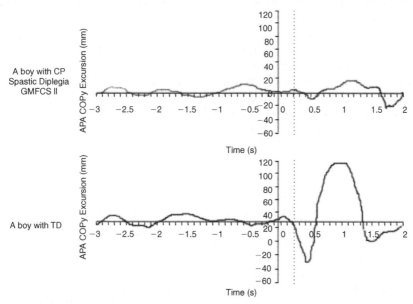

With this background on development of RPA and APA, what do we know about posture control of children with motor disabilities?

RPA AND APA IN CHILDREN WITH MOTOR DISABILITIES

The following section summarizes the research on RPA and APA of children with motor disabilities. Many studies have been completed on children with CP, with few studies on children with other motor disabilities. Details on each study referenced are listed in Table 2 for RPA and Table 3 for APA for the reader's further examination of sample and methodology.

RPA in Children with Cerebral Palsy

Because cerebral palsy (CP) is a neuromuscular impairment caused by non-progressive single or multiple lesions in the immature brain prior to, during or shortly after birth, motor impairments and possible sensory deficits may be present (Olney & Wright, 2000; Scherzer & Tschamuter, 1990). When considering the child with CP the areas of the body (monplegia, diplegia, hemiplegia, quadriplegia) must be considered, as well as, possible muscle tone abnormalities according to the area of the central nervous system affected (spasticity, ataxia, athetosis). The severity of the problem in terms of the effect on gross motor mobility should also be considered. The Gross Motor Function Classification System (GMFCS) rates children as: Level 1–walks without assistance but unable to keep up with peers, Level 2–walks without assistance but falls, and Level 3–walks with assistive devices, Level 4–primary mobility by wheelchair with moderate assistance, Level 5–needs full assistance for mobility in wheelchair (Palisano, Rosenbaum, Walter et al., 1997). Postural control issues have been investigated in children with different diagnoses and categories of CP.

FIGURE 5. Reactive postural adjustments studied in children as development of *sensory adaptation* to conditions of intersensory conflict. The child stands on a platform apparatus where the standing surface and or a visual surround is sway referenced to match the sway of the subject. Six sensory conditions are: 1) eyes open with firm surface (no sensory conflict), 2) eyes closed with firm surface (no vision), 3) firm surface with visual surround sway referenced (inaccurate visual information), 4) eyes open with sway referenced surface (inaccurate somatosensory information), 5) eyes closed with sway referenced surface (vestibular sensation only inaccurate visual and somatosensory information) and 6) visual surround and surface sway referenced (vestibular sensation only within accurate visual and somatosensory information) (Adapted from Horak, Shumway-Cook & Black, 1988)

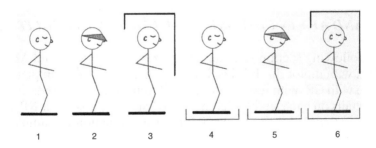

1   2   3   4   5   6

TABLE 2. Summary of Studies Examining RPA Postural Control in Children with Disabilities

Reference by Disability	Sample Composition & Size (N)	Age in Years	Testing Protocol (RPA, APA)	Measurements	Areas of Postural Control Impairment: (Sensory [S], Motor [Mo], Musculoskeletal [Mu])
Cerebral Palsy (CP)					
Brogen, Hadders-Algra & Forssberg, 1998	10 with mild to severe spastic diplegia and 10 matched controls	4 - 11	RPA in sitting in crossed leg position with platform perturbations	EMG of neck, trunk, hip flexor and extensor muscles	Mo - RPA reversals [cephalo-caudal muscle activation], simultaneous activation of ventral muscles, excessive co-contractions
Brogen, Forssberg, & Hadders-Algra, 2001	10 with mild to severe spastic diplegia and 10 matched controls	3 - 7.5	RPA in sitting in erect vs. crouched sitting posture with platform perturbations	EMG of neck, trunk, & hip muscles Kinematics of head, body sway and pelvis	Mu - Mechanical configuration of a crouched posture provided a solution to instability in sitting.
Nashner, Shumway-Cook & Marin, 1983	10 with CP (3 each with spastic hemiplegia, spastic diplegia & ataxia; 1 with athetosis), and 10 matched control children	7 - 9	- RPA in standing with platform perturbations - RPA in standing with 6 sensory conflict conditions	- EMG of leg, thigh and trunk muscles - Forceplates to measure sway trajectories in torque traces	Mo, Mu - Children with *spasticity*: delayed muscle onsets latencies, reversals - Children with ataxia: longer onset latencies S - Children with ataxia had increased sway and often lost balance
Ferdjallah, Harris, Smith, & Wertsch, 2002	11 ambulatory children with spastic diplegia, 8 control children	CP: 5-18 Control: 5-13	RPA in standing eyes open and closed	Forceplates for sway by COP measures	Mu - Children with CP had transverse rotation control for balance
Rose, Wolff, Jones, Bloch, Oehlert & Gamble, 2002	23 ambulatory children with spastic diplegia, 92 control children	5 - 18	RPA in standing eyes open and closed	Forceplates for sway by COP measures	Mu - Children with CP had increased path length, mean radial displacement, and diffusion coefficient than control children
Burtner, Qualls & Woollacott, 1998; Woollacott, Burtner, Jensen et al., 1998	7 with spastic diplegia; 7 controls matched in walking experience	1.7 - 14	RPA in crouched standing with platform perturbations	EMG of leg, thigh and trunk muscles	Mo, Mu - Controls showed nonselective activation of agonist vs. antagonist muscles, & reversals similar to children with spasticity
Bai, Bertenthal & Sussman, 1987	1 with ataxic CP and 3 controls	3	RPA during moving room visual flow	Videotape & behavioral coding of postural responses	S - Child with ataxia staggered or fell on most trials; Controls did not

TABLE 2 (continued)

Reference by Disability	Sample Composition & Size (N)	Age in Years	Testing Protocol (RPA, APA)	Measurements	Areas of Postural Control Impairment: (Sensory [S], Motor [Mo], Musculoskeletal [Mu])
Liao, Jeng, Lai, Cheng, & Hu, 1997	8 with spastic diplegia CP, 16 controls	5-12	RPA in standing with 6 sensory conflict conditions	Forceplates to measure COP displacements	S - Children with CP with decreased stability also had slower gait velocity & increased physiological cost
Lowes, 1997; Westcott, Lowes, Richardson, Crowe & Deitz, 1997	35 with CP; 24 with spastic diplegia, 8 with hemiplegia, 3 with quadriplegia	6-14	Pediatric Clinical Test of Sensory Interaction for Balance (PCTSIB); six sensory conditions tested using foam & dome	Time & sway in each position, transformed into ordinal categories, & then into sensory condition categories	S - Children with hemiplegia showed no problems with sensory interaction - Children with diplegia showed significant differences between somatosensory accurate and inaccurate categories
Down Syndrome (DS)					
Shumway-Cook & Woollacott, 1985b	6 with DS 11 age matched controls	1-6	RPA in standing posture with platform perturbations	EMG of leg, thigh and trunk muscles	Mo, Mu - Children with DS had delayed muscle onsets in proximal muscles & instability at knee & hip
Kokubun Shinyo, Ogita et al., 1997	11 with DS & 17 with other MR	DS: 10-19 MR: 13-18	RPA Standing posture	Forceplate to measure COP displacement, head sway	Mu - Greater sway in one foot standing balance
Westcott, Lowes, Richardson, Crowe, & Deitz, 1997	9 with Down syndrome	4-12	PCTSIB; six sensory conditions tested using foam & dome	Time & sway in each position, transformed into ordinal categories, & then into sensory condition categories	S - More sway and less time in conditions with absent visual input
Developmental Coordination Disorder					
Horak, Shumway-Cook, Crowe & Black, 1988	30 with hearing loss; 15 with LD & motor clumsiness (DCD); & 54 controls	7-11	RPA in standing with 6 sensory conflict conditions	Potentiometer to measure sway	S - Children with DCD had difficulty with balance in conditions of sensory conflict
Smyth & Mason, 1998	146 who were right handed; 73 with DCD, & 73 controls	5-8	RPA in clinical tests of motor function	Kinesthetic Sensitivity Test & Movement ABC	S, Mo - Children with DCD lower performance in complex motor tasks and balance, not just due to poor proprioception

TABLE 2 (continued)

Reference by Disability	Sample Composition & Size (N)	Age in Years	Testing Protocol (RPA, APA)	Measurements	Areas of Postural Control Impairment: (Sensory [S], Motor [Mo], Musculoskeletal [Mu])
Deitz, Richardson, Westcott, & Crowe, 1996	72 children: 36 with LD and motor in-coordination, 36 with typical development	6-9	RPA in standing with 6 sensory conflict conditions	Sway and time in conditions on the P-CTSIB	S - Children with LD significantly lower balance scores in vision absent, vision inaccurate, somatosensory inaccurate, and vestibular only conditions.
Hearing Impairment (HI)					
Horak, Shumway-Cook, Crowe, & Black, 1988	30 with HI; 15 with LD & motor clumsiness; & 54 control children	7-11	RPA in standing with 6 sensory conflict conditions	Potentiometer to measure sway	S - Children with HI had difficulty with balance in conditions that required only vestibular information
Selz, Girardi, Konrad, & Hughes, 1996	15 with congenital or acquired HI before the age of 2 yrs	8-17	Ocular movements	Electronystag-mography during positional & rotation tests	S - Vestibular differences in both groups; may be related to balance disorders
Casselbrandt, Redfern, Fruman, Fall, & Mandel, 1998	11 with otitis media with effusion & 11 age matched controls	3-9	RPA Optic flow conditions	High and low stimulus conditions	S - Children with OME had greater sway velocity than control children
Prenatal exposure to toxins					
Roebuck, Simmons, Richardson, Mattson & Riley, 1998	12 with alcohol exposure and 12 age/ sex matched controls	8-16	RPA Rapid toes up platform movements	EMG of triceps surae and anterior tibialis muscles	S - AE Children had over reliance on somatosensory information (increased sway when visual & vestibular information unavailable)
Bhattacharya, Shukla, Dietrich, Bornschein & Berger, 1995	162 with high lead concentration in blood	6	RPA Standing maintenance	Forceplate to measure sway	Mu - Children had increased variable sway and poor balance

RPA OF CHILDREN WITH SPASTIC CP IN SITTING

Results of sitting perturbation studies (Brogen, Hadders-Algra, & Forssberg, 1998) suggest that the children with CP have disordered muscle activations (RPA reversals [cephalo-caudal muscle activation], simultaneous activation of ventral muscles, excessive co-contractions) for sitting postural control. Interestingly, the sitting position of the child

TABLE 3. Summary of Studies Examining APA Postural Control in Children with Disabilities

References by Disability	Sample Composition & Size (N)	Age	Testing Protocol (RPA, APA)	Measurements	Areas of Postural Control Impairment: (Sensory [S], Motor [Mo], Musculoskeletal [Mu])
Cerebral Palsy (CP)					
Hadders-Algra, van der Fits, Stremmelaar, & Touwen, 1999	7 high-risk infants, 5 went on to develop spastic hemiplegia, 1 spastic tetraplegia, & 1 spastic tetratplegia & atheosis	Corrected ages 3-10 months	APA, Reaching was elicited in 4 positions: lying supine, sitting semi-reclined, upright sitting, & 'long-leg' sitting	Videotaped analysis for onset & velocity of reach, position of trunk & pelvis @ reach, & qualitative assessment of goal-directed movement; EMG onsets & amplitudes of deltoid & APA; patterns of APA	Mo & S - 6 infants with spastic CP had basic APA patterns, but later in development than typical; but had problems with modulating APA across different positions tested; authors hypothesized etiology to be both Mo & S - 1 infant with athetosis never showed basic APA or modulation across positions
Westcott, Zaino, Unanue, Thorpe, & Miller, 1998; Zaino & Westcott, 1997	54 children: 27 with spastic CP; 27 age matched with typical development (TD)	6-12 years	APA Stand and reach test; Timed Up and Go (TUG); Functional Reach Test (FRT); Running speed test (RS)	EMG onsets & motor coordination patterns (MCPs) of APA; scores on TUG, FRT, RS	Mo - Children with CP usually show similar patterns of APA, but slower reach, later APA onset times & greater variability than TD group - APA co-contraction use similar between children with CP & TD -no significant correlation of functional tests & APA MCPs in CP group
Liu, 2001	56 children: 28 with spastic CP, GMFCS Levels I & II; 28 age & gender matched with TD	4-12 years	APA Stand & reach test at slow & fast movement times	APA: EMG & COP onsets, amplitudes & patterns; Kinematics of reach and APA	Mo - spatial features of APA intact in children with CP, but slower reach times, direction-specific APA less consistent, onset of APA later, larger variability in temporal features & smaller modulation in quantitative parameters of APA, than in children with TD - walking experience, primary diagnosis, & GMFCS level related to APA

TABLE 3 (continued)

References by Disability	Sample Composition & Size (N)	Age	Testing Protocol (RPA, APA)	Measurements	Areas of Postural Control Impairment: (Sensory [S], Motor [Mo], Musculoskeletal [Mu])
Zaino, 1999	38 children: 19 with spastic CP, GMFCS Levels I & II; 19 age & gender matched children with TD	8-14 years	APA Stand & reach test	APA EMG and COP onset times and patterns	Mo -Children with CP show APAs with more distal posterior muscle onsets, decreased anterior-posterior COP pathlength & velocity, more medial-lateral excursion, increased medial-lateral pathlengths & velocity, & slower reach times, compared to TD group
Westcott, Zaino, Miller, Thorpe, Unanue, 1998	67 children: 32 with spastic CP, GMFCS Levels I, II, III; 35 with TD	6-12 years	APA Stand & reach test	APA EMG onset times & MCPs	Mo -Children with CP, GMFCS I, similar to children with TD - Children with CP, GMFCS II & III, different APA MCPs than Level I or TD group, showing earlier onset times for postural activity
Liu, Zaino, & Westcott, 2000	14 children: 7 with CP & GMFCS Level II, and 7 with TD	6-12 years	APA, Stand & reach test	APA - COP onset, amplitude and patterns	Mo -Children with CP had greater variability in the number of posterior COP APA excursions, & less variability in the medial-lateral COP APA excursions compared to TD group -Children with CP show earlier onsets of COP APA activity
Zaino & Westcott, 1997	28 children: 12 with spastic CP, 16 with TD	6-12 years	APA, Stand & reach	APA - EMG onset times & patterns	Mo - Children with CP had slower reach times, greater variability in APA patterns, minimal effects of learning across 10 trials, & less incidence of APA.
Thorpe, Zaino, Westcott & Valvano, 1998	16 with TD	6-12 years	APA, Stand & reach test from regular posture & from crouched posture	APA - EMG onset times & patterns	Mu -children in crouch position had more variability in the APA MCPs & were more likely to contract quadriceps sooner than in the regular stance position

TABLE 3 (continued)

References by Disability	Sample Composition & Size (N)	Age	Testing Protocol (RPA, APA)	Measurements	Areas of Postural Control Impairment: (Sensory [S], Motor [Mo], Musculoskeletal [Mu])
Zaino, Westcott, Miller, & Thorpe, 1997	36 children: 14 with spastic CP, 22 with TD	6-12 years	APA, stand and reach from firm & foam surfaces	EMG - APA onset times and patterns	Mo -all children showed variability, but children with CP had increased variability & use of co-contractions on foam surface
Down Syndrome (DS)					
Shumway-Cook & Woollacott, 1985b	17 children: 6 with DS, 11 controls	15 months - 6 years	APA, preparation for rotational floor perturbation across many trials	EMG - APA onset times of gastrocnemius muscle	Mo -children with DS did not attenuate APA across repeated trials as compared to attenuation in controls.
Developmental Coordination Disorder					
Fisher & Bundy, 1982	9 boys with LD & motor coordination dysfunction, 11 controls	LD group 6 - 9 years; TD group 4 - 11 years	Postural adjustments during a stand and reach as far as possible laterally	Scored kinematics of equilibrium postures during the task on a qualitative scale	Mo -children with LD showed less arm and leg counterbalancing & less distance reached compared to TD group
Myelomeningocele (MM)					
Norrlin, Karlsson, Ashlsten, Lanshammar, Silander, & Dahl, 2002	31 children: 11 with MM, 20 without physical impairment	10-13 years	APA, Rapid arm lift from the seated position in eyes open and closed conditions	APA COP changes were used to calculate COM acceleration and movement time	Mo - children with MM show lower sway frequency, & longer movement times than typical group - onset times of posterior APA COP shift were similar across the two groups

with CP may influence postural adjustments. When children with mild to moderate CP (children who were able to ambulate independently either with or without adaptive equipment) were perturbed in erect (crossed legs position, mean pelvic angle 89°) and crouched (legs positioned forward, mean pelvic angle 135°) sitting postures, the mechanical configuration of the crouched posture provided a solution to instability in sitting. These children were shown to be able to modulate their RPA

EMG activity in the crouch position, whereas they could not do this in the erect position. Thus the atypical *musculoskeletal* positioning used by these children improved their RPA postural responses (Brogen, Forssberg, & Hadders-Algra, 2001). The question remains, however, if the children performed better in the crouch position because the position offered something specific relative to the children's disability or if this is just the most practiced sitting position of children with mild to moderate CP, therefore, would potentially be the position where the child has learned the most adaptability.

RPA OF CHILDREN WITH CP IN STANDING

Motor processes differences have been noted specifically in the children with *spastic hemiplegia* with poor timing and delayed muscle onset latencies as well as reversal in muscle activation (proximal to distal sequencing rather than the expected distal to proximal pattern of muscle activation) in the legs with spasticity. Children with *ataxia* did not show these disordered patterns in muscle recruitment; however, they demonstrated longer onset latencies with trial to trial variations when compared with a control group of children without neuromuscular impairments (Nashner, Shumway-Cook, & Marin, 1983). The children with *spastic diplegia* CP were found not to have clear onsets and offsets of muscle activations and demonstrated prolonged durations of muscle activation. Children in the control group demonstrated a trend toward RPA characterized by a decrease in duration of muscle responses with increased walking experience, while children with spastic diplegia had RPA characterized by prolonged duration of muscle activation at all stages of stance and walking experience. The children with spastic diplegia showed nonselective activation of agonist and antagonist muscles, specifically they had: (a) increased frequency of reversals (proximal to distal recruitment of leg and thigh muscles); (b) increased recruitment of antagonist muscles; and (c) decreased activation of trunk musculature in response to platform perturbations (Burtner, Qualls, & Woollacott, 1998; Woollacott, Burtner, Jensen et al., 1998) (see Figure 6). Through examination of COP movement after perturbations, some children with CP showed greater COP displacement especially in a radial direction and slower frequencies of sway. A limb protraction/retraction control pattern was observed during medial-lateral sway and a transverse body rotation component during anterior-posterior sway as being effective strategies in both children with and without CP. The transverse rotation

FIGURE 6. Muscle activation in child's legs with and without spasticity following backward translation of the platform (vertical arrow). Note the reversal in muscle onset sequencing (horizontal arrows) in the leg with spasticity with hamstrings being activated prior to gastrocnemius (Adapted from Nashner, Shumway-Cook, & Marin, 1983)

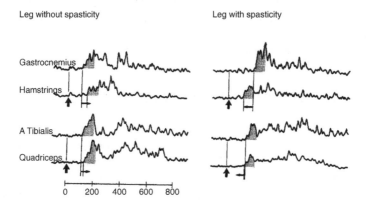

control contribution may be critical for postural stability in children with CP due to their overall relatively poor ankle control as compared to children without CP (Ferdjallah, Harris, Smith & Wertsch, 2002).

In terms of the *musculoskeletal* differences, when children with spastic diplegia adopt a crouched position (hips and knees flexed and ankles dorsiflexed) in stance, the musculoskeletal constraints (different starting position, as well as the presence of spasticity) affect their muscle recruitment during balance perturbation (Woollacott, Burtner, Jensen, Jasiewicz, Roncesvalles, & Sveistrup, 1998; Burtner, Woollacott, & Qualls, 1999).

When *sensory processes* were examined in children with ataxia, the studies suggest that visual dominant RPA are still present after 2 years age. However, it is unclear if the vision-dominant behavior was due to the presence of ataxia or delayed onset of walking (Bai, Bertenthal & Sussman, 1987). When sway responses of children with spastic and ataxic CP were analyzed in the six sensory conflict conditions, all children with CP had more sway than control children but the children with ataxia had the most difficulty and often had loss of balance (Nashner et al., 1983). On the clinical version of the Sensory Organization Test, the Pediatric Clinical Test of Sensory Interaction for Balance (P-CTSIB), children with spastic diplegia CP were found to have difficulty disregarding inaccurate somatosensory information (Lowes, 1997). Children with hemiplegia CP did not show any specific problems related to using sensory information for postural control.

RPA in Children with Other Motor Disabilities

Delayed muscle onsets in the proximal muscles characterized the RPA of children with Down syndrome (DS). This leads to biomechanical consequences of excessive motion at the knee and hip with resultant postural instability (Shumway-Cook & Woollacott, 1985b; Woollacott & Shumway-Cook, 1986). Further differentiation of the effects of low tone vs. cognitive deficits in this population were identified by Kokubun and colleagues (1997) who found greater sway in one foot standing balance in children with DS as compared to children with mental retardation (Kokubun Shinyo, Ogita et al., 1997). Using the P-CTSIB to examine sensory organization and use for postural control, Westcott and colleagues demonstrated that children with DS seem to have more difficulty balancing when visual input is eliminated (Westcott, Lowes, Richardson, Crowe, & Deitz, 1997). These children continue to rely on vision as their primary input for postural control long after typically developing children would mature out of this.

Sensory organization differences are often present in children with Developmental Coordination Disorder (DCD). Children with learning differences and DCD had greater body sway than typically developing children in all conflict balance conditions (visual, somatosensory [cutaneous and proprioception], and vestibular) as well as decreased scores on the Bruininks-Oseretsky Test of Motor Proficiency–Balance subscale (Horak, Shumway-Cook, Crowe & Black, 1988). Deitz and colleagues (1996) also tested children with learning disabilities and motor in-coordination on the P-CTSIB (Deitz, Richardson, Westcott, & Crowe, 1996). They demonstrated similar results in that the children with motor disability scored significantly lower on the sensory conflict conditions than typical age-matched peers. Although the individual contribution of proprioception to balance and motor performance difficulties has been investigated in 5-8 year old children with DCD, the children's decreased performance was found to be related to many features of complex motor tasks, not just poor proprioception (Smyth & Mason, 1998).

Children with hearing impairments have been found to have difficulties with RPA when reliance on vestibular information alone was available for balance (conditions 5 & 6 of the Sensory Organization Test) (Horak et al., 1988). The vestibular differences in this population appear to be present in children with congenital and acquired hearing loss at an early age (Selz, Girardi, Konrad & Hughes, 1996). The effect of transient factors on auditory/vestibular functions was also explored in children with otitis media with effusion (OME) in conditions of optic flow to challenge their balance (Casselbrandt, Redfern, Fruman, Fall, & Mandel, 1998). Results suggested that children with OME were more visually dependent than age matched control children for balance maintenance due to vestibular sensory differences.

Children who have been exposed prenatally to alcohol often display impaired fine and gross motor skills including balance maintenance. These children display over reliance on somatosensory information for balance control with increased sway when visual and vestibular information was not available (Roebuck, Simmons, Richardson, Mattson & Riley, 1998). Increased postural sway as measured by a force platform system has also been observed in children who have been chronically exposed to lead. The lead is thought to have an effect on the proprioception sensory system. Postural sway deficits in this population were not related to socio-economic, racial or other environmental factors (Bhattacharya, Shukla, Dietrich, Bornschein & Berger, 1995).

APA in Children with Cerebral Palsy

A longitudinal study of APA *motor processes* during a sit and reach task was completed in infants with CP (Hadders-Algra, van der Fits, Stremmelaar, & Touwen, 1999). Six infants, who at an older age were diagnosed to have spastic CP, displayed the basic developmental components of typical postural control in sitting, but did so at ages older than those of typically developing infants. These infants, however, had difficulty modulating their responses based on specific task and environmental constraints. Both motor coordination and sensory integration problems were hypothesized to cause these limitations. The infant who developed spasticity and athetosis was never able to show the basic components of trunk postural control in sitting and had a great deal of variability in the postural activations which did not seem to decrease with age.

In a stand and reach task, children with and without cerebral palsy showed variability in the postural motor coordination patterns used with anticipatory activity occurring in most children (Westcott, Zaino, Unanue, Thorpe & Miller, 1998). However, there was more variability in the motor coordination patterns used by the children with CP (Liu, 2001; Westcott, Zaino, Unanue et al., 1998; Zaino, 1999). The children specifically showed a greater incidence of distal posterior muscle onsets initially (gastrocnemius), as compared to the more typical pattern of anterior muscles first (anterior tibialis) (Zaino, 1999); and the amplitude of the APA EMG activity was smaller than typical (Liu, 2001). When classified on the GMFCS (Palisano et al., 1997), the children at the highest functional level (level 1) showed more similar postural motor coordination patterns to children without CP (Westcott, Zaino, Miller, Thorpe, & Unanue, 1998). The children in GMFCS level 2 with greater practice began to approach the patterns used by the typical children. Temporal features of the EMG patterns showed the most variability, specifically showing slower onset times and larger times between the onset of the APA and the onset of the reach (Liu, 2001). The children in GMFCS level 3, while showing some similarities in terms of postural motor coordination patterns, were very variable. These children showed the *earliest* activation of anticipatory postural muscle contractions, an average of approximately 400 msec prior to arm movement (monitored by anterior deltoid contraction) as compared to approximately 60 msec for typical and GMFCS level 1(Westcott, Zaino, Miller et al., 1998). This may be a compensatory mechanism where the child must prepare well in advance for the internal perturbation caused by the reaching maneuver, i.e., they may be using postural preparations rather than APAs (see Figure 1). As a consequence, the postural control and the prime movement of reaching may not be synchronized temporally resulting in poor coordination of the movement (Westcott, Zaino, Miller et al., 1998; Liu, 2001).

Our research (Westcott and colleagues) suggests that when reaching, children with CP demonstrate compensatory strategies to keep the movement of the body's COG well within the BOS. Children with CP appear to move their center of pressure under their feet more in a medial-lateral direction (increased COP path length) and less in the anterior-posterior direction than do children with typical development while reaching forward (Liu, Zaino, & Westcott, 2000; Zaino, 1999). Excursions of their COP movement also are smaller, meaning that they do not move their COP as far as the typically developing group (see Figure 4). As well, the onset time and velocity of the postural adjustment during the reach is variable and decreased in children with CP. As compared to children with typical development, the reaching maneuver in children with CP is slower and shorter when asked to reach the maximal distance possible (Liu, 2001; Zaino, 1999; Zaino & Westcott, 1997). When instructed to reach more quickly or to reach for a ball that is moving towards them, children with CP did show some modulation in their reaching time and the APA (Liu, 2001). However, based on the variability of the responses, overall the children with CP still seem to be searching for the appropriate APA strategy to use. These differences may be due to altered musculoskeletal or sensory experiences or just decreased experience in standing, walking, and reaching quickly as the children who had the longest walking experience demonstrating slightly better APA control (Liu, 2001).

In terms of *musculoskeletal* effects during APA, in agreement with the studies noted above (Woollacott et al., 1998; Burtner et al., 1999), when children with typical development were asked to reach forward from a crouched standing position, the motor coordination patterns used became more like those of age and gender matched children with CP who were in a crouched position, i.e., more APA variability and use of co-contraction activity (Thorpe, Zaino, Westcott, & Valvano, 1998). Therefore again, although there are neurological differences that affect postural control, musculoskeletal differences which lead to altered biomechanical resting postures add to the dysfunction.

Examination of *sensory processes* during tasks involving measurement of APA has been completed by having children perform the stand and reach task from different types of floor surfaces. Children with CP showed more difficulty with the stand and reach task on foam and beam surfaces as compared to a firm surface, and used more variable APA motor coordination patterns than children with typical development (Zaino, Westcott, Miller & Thorpe, 1998). The children with CP also did not show as much of a learning process, evidenced by reduced variability of APA coordination patterns, across 10 trials as did the typically developing group.

In summary, it appears that children with CP who are able to walk and have more movement experience have the basic innate APA patterns, however, they are not very successful with modulation or adaptation of these basic patterns to varying task and environmental conditions. Children with greater functional movement ability, appear more successful in learning to modulate APA. Children with more involvement appear to adopt alternative less efficient and variable strategies including proximal to distal contractions and co-contractions. Or they may also learn to either prepare their posture well in advance of a goal directed movement and/or adopt alternative goal directed movement patterns in order to not challenge postural control to any great extent. It appears that musculoskeletal changes (i.e., changes in range of motion in the hip/knee/ankle) causing adoption of different static positions affect APA motor patterns to a certain extent, especially related to increasing co-contraction of muscle groups. Children with CP show more variability when the sensory conditions of a task are changed, perhaps indicating that they are not utilizing sensory information as well as children with typical development.

APA in Children with Other Motor Disabilities

To date only Shumway-Cook and Woollacott (1985b) have examined an aspect of APA in children with DS. They documented that children with DS used APA in advance of a rotational platform perturbation which caused a quick plantar flexion at the ankle. Across repeated trials, this APA attenuated in children with typical development of comparable age as is seen in adults. The children with DS did not show an adaptation of this response. Shumway-Cook and Woollacott (1985b) suggest that the delay in the long-latency reflex and cerebellar pathology in individuals with DS may account for these results. Several studies on adults with Down syndrome may also give insight into the APA issues in children. Six individuals with Down syndrome, mean age 24.8 years, were asked during standing to flex and extend their arms quickly while EMG was recorded from the lower extremity muscles (Aruin & Almedia, 1997). These individuals showed anticipatory activity but used co-activation of the agonist-antagonist pairs of muscle as their postural strategy. The researchers hypothesized that this was an adaptive strategy used as the optimal way for these individuals to maintain control. In all movements, people with DS have been shown to use a greater amount of co-contraction of agonist/antagonist muscles, perhaps as an adaptation to limitations in control of individual joints, and slower movement times perhaps to overcome the lower resting muscle tone and less sensitive proprioceptive sensation integration.

Based on one study of APA using a stand and lateral reach protocol, it has been demonstrated that boys with learning disorders and motor in-coordination (DCD) counter balance when reaching laterally with less arm and leg abduction and extension than children without DCD. Their movements also appeared stiffer. These children may be restricting the movement of their center of gravity projection to small areas under the BOS (i.e., not reaching as far) and stiffening or freezing their degrees of freedom in order to improve stability (Fisher & Bundy, 1982).

Recently, postural control during a voluntary arm movement from a sitting position has been examined in children with myelomeningocele (Norrlin, Karlsson, Ashlsten et al., 2002). The children with myelomeningocele were found to move slower and to have a slower sway frequency as compared to the typical group. This slower movement was not related to the myelomeningocele level, therefore was hypothesized to be associated with other central nervous system differences in the children.

Summary of Postural Control in Children with Motor Disabilities

It is apparent that postural control is a complex motor behavior and children with motor disabilities and different diagnoses show a variety of problems. While it is interesting and somewhat helpful to look at different types of disabilities/diagnoses to determine general problems with postural control by diagnosis group, it also becomes apparent that each child needs to be examined individually to determine what his/her specific postural control problems are. A thorough examination and interpretation of findings is critical to the development of appropriate intervention plans. Readers are directed to recent reviews and studies of possible tests and measures for examination of postural control (Corriveau, Hebert, Prince, & Raiche, 2000; Gill, Allum, Carpenter, Held-Ziolkowska, Adkin, Honegger, & Pierchala, 2001; Kembhavi, Darrah, Magill-Evans, & Loomis, 2002; Shumway-Cook & Woollacott, 1993; Westcott, 2001; Westcott, Richardson, & Lowes, 1997).

INTERVENTION TO IMPROVE POSTURAL CONTROL IN CHILDREN

Evidence to direct intervention can come from indirect sources including the studies noted above examining the development of postural control in children with typical development, and studies examining the differences in postural control of children with motor disabilities. But intervention effectiveness studies provide the most directly applicable evidence to guide practice. The intervention studies designed to improve postural control in children summarized below are categorized as much as possible as either: (1) Handling and manipulation of the child by the therapist, in order to use sensory input to evoke postural control (i.e., to improve RPA), and (2) Activities where the therapist directs the task and environment and requires practice of active movement, forcing the child to create his own optimal pattern of goal directed postural control accompanying movement (i.e., to improve APA). Many interventions, however, can be a combination of both. Interventions related to practice of movement versus those directed at remediation of potential *rate-limiting* deficits/problems in the individual systems coordinating to produce postural control are also delineated. Finally, we have separated the studies demonstrating changes on typically developing children from those using children with disabilities.

Intervention to Change Postural Control in Typically Developing Children

Facilitation of postural control in typically developing children may provide insight into intervention for children with developmental differences. Four recent studies are highlighted. Use of additional postural support via adaptive equipment is a common intervention for children with postural instability. In 6-month-old infants who were not yet able to sit, it has been demonstrated that the use of a modified chair, giving better postural support at the hips and legs improves head stability and reaching behaviors (Hopkins & Ronnqvist, 2002). Designing practice of motor skills is another common intervention used by occupational and physical therapists. Two studies have investigated the effects of massed practice on the development of RPA in typically developing infants. Hadders-Algra, Brogen, and Forssberg (1996a; 1996b) investigated the effect of sitting balance training over a period of two months and found that postural response modulation increased with intervention (toy presentation in the border zone of reaching without falling, i.e., provoking APA). In a second study, Sveistrup and Woollacott (1997) investigated effects of massed practice experience on the development of stance postural responses in infants at the pull-to-stand stage of development. When comparing infants in the practice group (300 platform perturbations within a three day window of time, i.e., provoking RPA) to control infants on pre- and post-test measures, no differences in onset latencies were noted, however infants in the practice group showed an increase in the probability of muscle responses and better temporal organization.

Practice of quick reaching from standing across 10-20 trials was found to alter the APA in typically developing children, age 6-14 years. The APA decreased in variability, especially when the stand and reach activity was completed from a compliant versus firm surface (Zaino, 1999; Zaino et al., 1998). Practice of stand and reach with the addition of wrist weights in children 9-14 years with typical development was also found to reduce the variability in the APA and to specifically decrease the amplitude of the anterior-posterior APA COP movement prior to the reach onset (Zaino, Westcott, Ideishi, & Gocha, 1999).

Intervention for Improving Postural Control in Children with Motor Disabilities

Interventions for RPA

A recent study (Shumway-Cook, Woollacott, Hutchinson, Kartin, & Price, submitted) suggests positive effects of massed practice of RPA during platform perturbation (100 perturbations/day for 5 days with perturbations being 3-6 cm translation forward and backward that randomly ranged from 12cm/s to 24 cm/s) in 7-13 year old children with spastic diplegia and spastic hemiplegia. Using a single-subject multiple-baseline experimental design, all children demonstrated a significant improvement in their RPA (reduced COP area and time to stabilization) following the training program and 30 days post intervention. Thus, RPA postural control mechanisms of school-aged children with CP appear to be modifiable.

Providing a perturbation that the child is to resist, or passively assisting the child to weight shift in different positions are commonly used interventions to improve postural control (Westcott, Hartzler-Murray, & Pence, 1998). Weight shifting can be accompanied by various forms of facilitation and inhibition techniques as advocated by Bobath, Brunnstrom, Rood, and Voss, in order to have the resultant movement produced in a more effective fashion (Daldeiden, 1990; Shumway-Cook & McCullom, 1991). Evaluation of the overall effectiveness of the NDT approach used today which incorporates many techniques described by Bobath and Rood have shown only small changes in the motor outcomes measured with a specific deficit in studies related to potential changes in postural adjustment (Butler & Darrah, 2001). It is generally thought that while we can make differences in posture and movement when we have our hands on the child, the carry over to use of these patterns in general functional movement is questionable (Horak, 1992). A randomized controlled study examined the use of NDT techniques to improve postural control and movement in premature infants at high risk for developmental disability (Girolami & Campbell, 1994). This study showed a positive outcome of improved postural control in the treated group versus the control group. This study suggests that early NDT treatment is effective for improving postural muscle tone, but the question remains as to how long the effect lasts and if the improvements in postural control also lead to improvements in functional motor skill development.

Horseback riding as therapeutic practice of responding to constant perturbations in sitting was shown to improve static standing postural alignment of children with CP (Bertoti, 1988). Unfortunately, dynamic postural stability control was not examined as an outcome. More recently, it has been demonstrated that with use of horseback riding and hippotherapy techniques, children with CP improved their trunk posture, energy expenditure during gait, and showed better walking, running, and jumping ability (MacPhail, Edwards, Golding et al., 1998; McGibbon, Andrade, Widener, & Cintas, 1998). Kuezynski and Slonka (1999) tested artificial saddle riding effects on postural control in children with CP. Through a 3 month intervention including artificial saddle riding for 20 minutes twice a week, they found that the postural sway COP range, standard deviation, average speed and radius all decreased with the treatment. Butler (1998) tested a similar idea in 6 children with CP who at the beginning of the intervention were unable to sit without support. Each child was positioned on a rocking chair which supported the trunk. The seating device provided support to trunk and hip joints to the level where control was not automatic. When automatic postural control was attained at the targeted level, the supports were lowered. The children sat in the chair for 20 minutes −2.5 hours/day, 5-7 times per week, for 12-25 weeks. Perturbations were provided to the chair at periodic but unsuspected times to the child. All children were reported to attain independent sitting balance after completion of the intervention. The author utilized a specific testing procedure, for which she demonstrated inter-rater reliability, to determine the level of the trunk supports and to score independent sitting.

Butler and colleagues (1992) also examined the effects of ankle foot orthoses (AFO) and practice of RPA in 6 children with CP using a pre-test, post-test group design (Butler, Thompson, & Major, 1992). The children were 3-6 years-old and able to stand and walk independently, but displayed excessive plantar flexion, knee hyperextension, hyperflexion of the hip, and increased lumbar lordosis during gait. The intervention consisted of perturbations given to the children when in kneel standing. The child was not allowed to recover balance using hands for hip stabilization in order to focus the control at the knees. The kneel-perturbation exercise was completed for 10-15 minutes a session, 5-7 times/week, for 4-6 months. Solid ankle AFOs were adjusted using ground reaction force monitoring to bring the ground reaction force vector as close as possible to normal alignment at the knee. AFOs were worn throughout the day, seven days per week. Through gait analysis, Butler reported a reduction in the knee-extending moment arm in all limbs, improved foot/ground contact in three limbs, and improved balance in kneeling and ankle balance reactions in half of the children.

Interventions for APA

Active weight shifting in a rocking or repetitive manner is thought to encourage equilibrium responses and to give the patient the appropriate practice in balancing (Daldeiden, 1990). Following the systems theory of motor control, if APA is impaired, weight shifting should be done actively and it should be incorporated in a functional activity rather than practiced in isolation (Shumway-Cook & McCollum, 1991). Winstein and colleagues conducted an intervention effectiveness study of practice with weight shifting on a force platform with computer feedback in *adults* with hemiplegia (Winstein, Gardner, McNeal, Barto, & Nicholson, 1989). After treatment, the adults improved significantly compared to controls in their ability to weight shift on the platform, but did not improve their weight shift during their gait pattern. Weight-shift practice on a similar apparatus was examined in four children with CP using a case study design (Hartveld & Hegarty, 1996). Variable results were found with two of the children showing consistent improved ability to weight shift on the apparatus. No functional movement outcome was measured. This suggests that active weight shift can be improved by practice with feedback or knowledge of results about performance. However, long term carryover during daily activities has not been demonstrated.

Researchers examining the effects of practice of particular postural control activities have shown consistently that improvement in the practiced motor behavior will occur. Effgen showed that with practice of one foot balance and other narrow stance positions, children with hearing impairment improved significantly in their ability to stand on one foot (Effgen, 1981). However, this did not decrease the children's standing sway as measured on a force plate system. Practice of more general movements to improve postural control has shown mixed outcomes. There has been significant postural improvement in some studied groups of children and non-significant improvement in others (Horvat, 1982; Boswell, 1991; Lewis, Higham, & Cherry, 1985). Recently in children with DS, the practice of jumping was examined in terms of changes in quality of jumping skill, and scores on the Bruininks-Oseretesky Test of Motor Proficiency–Balance subscale (Wang & Chang, 1997). While improvements on the total score of the balance subtests were found, no significant change was seen in one foot floor or beam stand or the floor heel to toe walk. All these results may be reflective of the specificity of training effect related to practice.

RATE-LIMITING SYSTEMS INTERVENTION

Musculoskeletal Intervention

Strength Intervention with Children with CP. Studies which have approached changing the *musculoskeletal* status of children with CP, specifically force production capability, have not routinely examined outcomes related specifically to postural control, but have examined the children for changes in gait control (Damiano, Kelly & Vaughan, 1995; Damiano, Vaughan, & Abel, 1995; Wiley & Damiano, 1998). Children with CP can, with regular strengthening exercise programs, improve their force production capability. But there are mixed results as to whether this improves the gait pattern and possibly postural control during gait (Wiley & Damiano, 1998). The mixed results probably stem from the individual problems or constraints that each child with CP has (Westcott & Lowes, 1995). Preliminary results of a study examining the effects of a 6 week weight training program with 3 school-aged individuals with spastic diplegia (7-22 years) suggest the intervention has positive effects on balance, gait and functional skills. Changes in RPA reported in these children were increased balance maintenance during platform translations of greater size and speed in two subjects and an increased use of ankle strategies to maintain balance in two children post intervention. Peak joint angles (ROM) during gait more closely approximated typically developing children post strength training suggesting more normalized motor control during walking. Significant changes in activities requiring balance were also reported as measured by three subtests of the School Function Assessment (Philips, 2002; Schlosser, Philips & Burtner, 2002).

Use of Ankle-Foot Orthoses. Lower extremity casting, splinting, or ankle foot orthoses, have been examined in terms of effectiveness in altering postural control in standing in children with CP and DCD (Anderson, Snow, Dorey et al., 1988; Bertoti, 1986; Embrey, Yates, & Mott,1990; Harris & Riffle, 1986; Hinderer, Harris, Purdy et al., 1988; Orner, Turner, Worrell, 1994; Radtka, Skinner, Dixon, Johanson, 1997; Watt, Sims, Harckham et al., 1986). Studies in the literature are single subject or repeated measures designs, with small numbers of subjects, often with no comparative control group. Significant improvement in standing postural control, gait stride length, and sometimes gait velocity have been the common outcomes. Use of dynamic splints that alter the movement coordination at the ankle joint less than occurs in fixed AFOs have shown positive results in three studies. Embrey, Yates, and Mott

(1990), in a single-subject study, reported improvement in the knee joint control during walking with these splints. In a second study, the effect of ankle foot orthoses on balance was investigated in children with spastic diplegia and age matched typically developing children. During platform perturbations, both groups of children demonstrated muscle organization changes when solid AFOs were worn which included decreased recruitment of ankle musculature, disorganization of muscle response patterns, decreased use of ankle strategies and increased joint angular velocities at the knee as compared to balance responses when no or dynamic AFOs were worn (Burtner, Woollacott & Qualls, 1999). Rethlefsen et al. (1999) showed the best muscle patterns and gait with articulated AFOs, but only for those children who did not have a tendency to crouch (Rethlefsen, Kay, Dennis, Forstein, & Tolo, 1999). Another study suggests no differences in motor coordination comparing dynamic splints to standard solid AFOs (Radtka et al., 1997). The effect of improved postural control in standing and in gait with the AFOs seems to be immediate but not to carry over when the AFOs are removed (Harris & Riffle, 1986; Radtka et al., 1997). These studies suggest preventing or modifying plantar flexion in children with motor disabilities, has benefits for postural control. This may be because of an increased BOS from the foot flat position. The extra weight of the AFO and the lack of need to control the ankle degrees of freedom may also be the reason for postural control improvement. More research is needed to determine the reasons for improvement and what type of concomitant therapy intervention might enhance carry-over of improved postural and movement control when the child is not wearing the AFO.

Sensory Intervention

Research on *sensory* stimulation to cue individuals to respond with appropriate postural adjustments is sparse and primarily involves direct stimulation of the vestibular system by spinning and/or quick start and stop linear movement (Chee, Kreutzberg, & Clark, 1978; Gabert, Jee, & Collins, 1982; Zimmerman, Gross, & Speckhart, 1993). Improvements in postural control were observed in these children after the treatment, but long term carry-over to functional activity was not examined. Children with sensorineural hearing loss and bilateral vestibular deficit were examined following a 12-week program (3 times/week) of sensory organization tasks for postural control. The children with this disability showed significant improvement in RPA. Specific changes in balance included: (a) increased ability to recruit the anterior tibialis muscle to maintain balance, (b) decreased postural sway during sensory conflict conditions, and (c) fewer stepping responses in the children in reaction to loss of balance (Rine, Spielholtz & Braswell, 2002).

Motor Intervention

Studies using primarily single subject or case study designs have examined changing the RPA and APA *motor processes* via the use of biofeedback devices to cue losses of head or trunk balance in sitting and foot positioning in walking. Improved performance has been documented after use of the augmented information even in children with severe physical and cognitive involvement (Bjork & Wetzel, 1983; Campbell, 1990). It has also been suggested based on a study of sitting balance in children who developed CP, that altering the position of the pelvis through seating devices and the addition of a weighted cuff during practice of reaching as a postural perturbation may provoke different adaptive RPA and APA, respectively (Hadders-Algra et al., 1999). Electrical stimulation has been used in children with CP to trigger activation of the dorsiflexors and plantarflexors during movement with some interesting changes in muscle coordination (Carmick, 1993, 1995). This intervention may be able to be applied to changing RPA or APA coordination. Finally, the use of various adaptive seating devices to provide support when postural control is lacking have improved postural alignment and potentially improved feeding and upper extremity motor control during sitting (Hulme, Shaver, Acher et al., 1987; Reid, 1996).

Almeida, Corcos, and Latash (1994), have demonstrated that with practice of fast arm movements (1,100 practice trials over 4 days) six *adult* subjects with DS, mean age 25 years, could learn to decrease co-contractions used in a reaching movement and instead use alternate agonist-antagonist contractions. Whether similar changes could occur in postural control coordination patterns with this amount of fast movement practice is unknown at the present time.

Summary of Intervention Research

There are a few types of intervention that have been shown to improve postural control in children. Based on *specificity of practice*, both RPA and APA can be improved in both typical and atypical children. The number of practices to demonstrate improvement range from 10-1100, therefore, therapists need to consider how this much practice can occur in a child's life. Overall the *musculoskeletal* interventions such as use of

AFOs, in particular AFOs with articulating ankles, demonstrate some positive movement changes, however, further research is needed to determine how and to what extent these interventions specifically change RPA or APA in children with disabilities. Studies on strengthening demonstrate that strength can be increased without increasing spasticity and may positively change RPA. We need to investigate the impact of increasing strength on the APA in children. The interventions to change *motor processes* have mixed results and the studies are based on small numbers of children. Use of RPA or APA practice, where the child problem solves the most adaptive solution for the task may be more productive than trying to impose a specific pattern of motor activity on a child. *Sensory* interventions have been generally positive in outcome including use of vestibular stimulation, augmented biofeedback, and one recent study examining practice of sensory organization tasks. Therapy that addresses the specific etiology of the problem or current *rate-limiting factors* within the child's systems coupled with tasks that are motivating to the child are probably critical to positive outcomes.

Campbell suggested in 1990, in relation to a review of the effectiveness of postural control intervention for children with cerebral palsy, that, "Although no truly conclusive evidence exists from well controlled studies of postural outcomes from physical therapy for CP, much suggestive data indicates the need for further documentation of these effects" (Campbell, 1990, p. 138). While more research has been conducted and we have a larger evidence base, further studies are required to fully understand outcomes. The focus of future research would be investigating specific results of practice within individual task/environment conditions in populations of children with motor disabilities and the relationship of the practice to the children's changes in their RPA and APA. Similarly, the relationship between documented changes in RPA and APA to positive changes in children's functional or recreational movement ability needs to be established, thereby showing evidence that the child's time and money were well spent.

IMPLICATIONS FOR PRACTICE AND FUTURE RESEARCH

Based on the evidence that currently exists in pediatric rehabilitation and following the systems theory of motor control, we are presenting an exploratory plan for intervention. These clinical suggestions and combinations of interventions will need to be examined experimentally to determine their effectiveness in different populations of children with specific postural disorders.

In general, intervention should be planned after a thorough clinical examination of the major systems necessary for RPA and for APA during movement. The first purpose of the examination is to determine the *rate-limiting factors* impeding postural control improvement. After the *rate-limiting factors* are potentially identified, then interventions to change these impairments of body structure or function can be implemented as part of the therapy. The second purpose of the examination is to determine what functional and recreational motor activities the child neeeds or wants to accomplish.

The intervention plan focuses on practice maintaining positions (static equilibrium) and controlling movement (dynamic equilibrium) that are related to the desired meaningful task for the child. The practice should be varied in terms of the environment in which it occurs and the way repetitions are specifically completed (massed vs. random practice) to teach generalization of the skill (Schmidt, 1988; Winstein, 1991). When practicing the task, the child may be assisted by asking him/her to cognitively problem solve the accomplishment of the task (Thorpe & Valvano, 2002) to assist in self-organization, and by including a great number of trials which include experience with failure (i.e., falls). The use of external feedback from the therapist through augmented information can be provided during the task to facilitate the child to try different movements (i.e., speeds of movements, movement with increased feedback/altered conditions via weights, altered surfaces, altered visual input, environment changes, etc.). Feedback in summary form, for instance verbally describing the success or failure of the child's practice of a movement, provided at intermittent times may also assist the child's learning.

The therapy session should begin with typical pre-exercise stretching/warm-up activities with the therapist utilizing facilitation and handling techniques from NDT as appropriate to the child. Use of NDT techniques is based upon the finding that these techniques have been shown to consistently assist with immediate improvement in range of motion, even though there have not been conclusive long term effects shown on range of motion (Butler & Darrah, 2001). The stretching would be followed with impairment of body structure/function intervention for *sensory, motor*, or *musculoskeletal rate-limiting factors*, and finally, for the majority of the session, practice of functionally meaningful movements under varied conditions. Evaluation of progress at the body structure/function level and at the functional activity level should be made periodically to determine the effectiveness of the program. Based on progress and ability of the child and family, the final outcome for the child and parent is for both the child and care-giver (until the child is old enough to handle it alone) to be able to control and implement the intervention relying on periodic episodes of physical or occupational therapy intervention when assistance is needed to problem solve movement solutions.

Specifically for postural control improvement, the interventions that follow, stem from the research evidence we have reviewed above. These ideas are summarized in Table 4.

(1) Musculoskeletal rate limiting factors:

(a) Passive stretching and joint mobilization techniques to increase joint and muscle range of motion should offer the child more options for a variety of motions especially in the ankle and the trunk to use for postural control. Based on studies of stretching collagen tissue in children with CP, the child may need to have prescribed environmental tasks that incorporate the available range of motion into his/her daily movement repertoire for at least 6 hours of the day (Tardieu, Tardieu, Colbeau-Justin, & Lespargot, 1982).

(b) Use of static orthoses can decrease recruitment of ankle musculature needed for ankle balance strategies while increasing the joint angular velocities at the knee. Since these changes were not present when dynamic AFOs were worn, this orthotic design is preferable if a child is able to practice and succeed at movement and balance when he has to use the ankle range and musculature. However, some children will require the additional mechanical support of solid AFOs to maintain balance as well as to correct and prevent deformities.

(c) Strengthening protocols to increase muscle torque capability and to improve ability to create a torque rapidly should be used if weakness is present. Preliminary results suggest that general strengthening programs assist in refinement of RPA, however, the control of muscle activations in smaller ranges of motion, in bursts of activation (quick contractions), and in functional positions/movements may be more beneficial than straight progressive resistive exercises.

(d) Seating devices to give assistance to upright postures need to be examined carefully dependent on the child's age, level of severity of the motor abnormality (for children with CP) and the focus of the activity to be completed from the sitting position. If the child is just relaxing, a slightly backward inclined position may be most appropriate. A more erect or slightly tilted forward position may better facilitate reach/grasp and practice active postural control.

TABLE 4. Summary of Exploratory Intervention Suggestions

Area of need for intervention	Passive interventions	Active interventions	Assistive devices
Musculoskeletal	- Passive stretch and joint mobilization to increase joint range over time - NDT techniques to loosen up joint range for the time of intervention (Butler & Darrah, 2001)	- Environmental/task adaptations to create need to use available joint range at least 6 hours/day (Tardieu et al., 1982) - Progressive resistive exercises (Damiano et al., 1995) - Active general movement with resistance, ex. pool exercise, movement with ankle weights, weighted vests, etc	- AFOs, prefer dynamic ankle joint (Burtner et al., 1999) - Seating devices, prefer more erect positioning, and position of slight anterior pelvic tilt
Motor		- Environmental/task modification to provoke ankle or hip strategy - Reaching to limits of stability - Reaching quickly (ex. to catch a ball) - Reach with weighted wrists (Bouisset et al., 2000) - Posture practice with augmented feedback	- Biofeedback on position via extra auditory, visual input - Use of AFOs - Adaptive seating devices
Sensory	- Provide increased sensory input (ex. swing/spin for vestibular)	- Environmental/task modifications to provoke use of a particular sense (vision, somatosensory, vestibular) - Training in complex motor activity to learn to shift from visual dominance to somatosensory dominance for postural control (Mesure et al., 1997)	
RPA practice		- Practice reacting to external perturbations (at least 10-1100 repetitions)(Sveistrup & Woollacott, 1997; Shumway-Cook et al., submitted)	
APA practice		- Practice which demands APA for success, ball throw/catch, jump, roller skate (Le Pellec & Maton, 1999, 2000, 2002; Shiratori & Latash, 2000, 2001) - Move as far as possible as fast as possible (Kaminski & Simpkins, 2001; Liu, 2001) - Decrease hand support (Slijper & Latash, 2000) - Decrease fear of falling via practice (Adkin et al., 2002)	
General balance practice		- Practice of activities of daily living - Practice of leisure/recreational motor activities of child's choice	

(2) Motor processes rate limiting factors:

(a) The environment and task can be modified to practice either producing the strategy not used (e.g., provoking use of an ankle strategy when a hip strategy is primarily used by the child via roller skating) or to provoke a more optimal strategy.

(b) Practice in reaching to the limits of stability and reaching quickly may be beneficial for children who actively use co-contractions and limit their movement speed and the distance they project their COG so as to not challenge stability. Reaching in reaction to an external stimulus (ball thrown to child) can be used to provoke faster reach movement and higher amplitude APA. This may be beneficial for children who have been found to move slowly, such as children with CP, DS, and myelomenigocele.

(c) Practice reaching with the hand weighted may provide increased proprioceptive information as well as potential strengthening; the duration of the APA may also increase with this type of practice (Bouisset, Richardson, & Zattara, 2000). But the use of wrist weights during reaching may cause the child to reduce the anterior-posterior COP movement, which for children with CP, may not be the desired outcome.

(d) Practice of posture and movement with feedback about the child's starting posture will affect the RPA and APA. This can be accomplished through use of mirrors, auditory input (bells, squeak toys), lights, or electrical stimulation to cue the child to change starting positions and thus the APA or RPA motor coordination pattern of the movement task. Adaptive equipment, chairs, AFOs, etc., can also assist, as detailed above.

(3) Sensory processes rate limiting factors:

(a) Practice in specific sensory environments to force the use of the underused sensory information or to exaggerate the input from a particular system is suggested. By gradually increasing the complexity of the sensory information, the child can be encouraged to practice sensory conflict resolution. This can be accomplished through dimming the lights or wearing fogged glasses to vary visual input, and by balancing/moving on foam surfaces, air-mattresses, rough ground, moveable surfaces, etc., to vary proprioceptive input.

(b) Providing an increased amount of sensory input (for instance, vestibular input) may also accentuate the use of the sensory pathways and improve sensory organization for better postural control. The question remains as to how much and how often this input may need to occur.

(c) Encouraging training in complex motor activities requiring postural control may assist with improving the child's ability to utilize somatosensory input for postural control. An adult study comparing untrained individuals to those who had trained in judo and classical dance, suggests that training results in a change from reliance on visual input to reliance on proprioception during unperturbed stance (Mesure, Amblard, & Cremieux, 1997).

(4) RPA and APA practice:

(a) To develop RPA, the child needs to practice reacting to external perturbations which stem from different sensory sources (surface moving, body being bumped, etc.). The number of practice trials to effect a change may be quite large, ranging from at least 10-1,100, based on typical adult, child, and atypical population studies noted above.

(b) To develop APA, the child needs to practice/explore movement which demands the use of APA for a successful outcome. Ball throw/catch, jumping, and roller skating have all been demonstrated in adult studies to require interesting use of APA and RPA (LePellec & Maton, 1999, 2000, 2002; Shiratori & Latash, 2000, 2001). Practice moving as far and as fast as possible may provoke a larger need for APA (Kaminski & Simpkins, 2001; Liu, 2001). In adults, it has also been shown that providing even small hand support during APA practice will alter the motor coordination pattern from lower extremity activity to upper extremity activity (Slijper & Latash, 2000), therefore, the use of hand support needs to be weighed against the outcome desired. Again as with the RPA, the amount of practice to cause change in the APA may be quite large.

(c) Practice postural control and movement with a decrease in the fear of movement and falling through practice in an environment that is safe and comfortable. Adkin and colleagues have shown in adults that the magnitude of APA increases when the fear of falling increases (Adkin, Frank, Carpenter, & Peysar, 2002). However, the child will need to experience "falling" in order to learn to adapt and change RPA and APA patterns so they are ultimately effective.

(5) Generalize balance practice to facilitate participation in social and cultural contexts:

(a) The child also needs motivation and assistance to practice new possible postural and primary movements in a regular environment. Practice of daily activities that challenge balance (reaching for clothes in closet, picking up toys from floor, carrying tray in cafeteria, increasing balance during showering and bathing activities) should be beneficial.

(b) Identification and practice of recreation activities of interest in which the child actively uses balance control should lead to better functional outcome. Activities with peers such as horseback riding, skiing, roller skating, tai chi (Wu, 2002), etc., have been shown or are suggested to be beneficial.

OVERALL CONCLUSIONS

More research needs to be done to improve our understanding of development of RPA and APA in children with and without disabilities and what interventions are most effective for changing RPA and APA in children with motor disabilities. However, based on the current knowledge, interventions to improve RPA and APA in children should include much practice within the context of a functional task or the behavior of interest. Interventions to modify or reduce musculoskeletal, motor, or sensory system impairments may assist with the child's improvement, but ultimately ability to change functional motor performance is the primary and most meaningful objective, therefore carry-over to functional and recreational movement must be incorporated into our intervention programs.

REFERENCES

Adkin, A. L., Frank, J. S., Carpenter, M. G., & Peysar, G. W. (2002). Fear of falling modifies anticipatory postural control. *Experimental Brain Research*, 143, 160-170.

Almeida, G. L., Corco, D. M., & Latash, M. L. (1994). Practice and transfer effects during fast single-joint elbow movements in individuals with Down syndrome. *Physical Therapy*, 74, 1000-1016.

Anderson, J. P., Snow, B., Dorey, F. J., & Kabo, J. M. (1988). Efficacy of soft splints in reducing severe knee-flexion contractures. *Developmental Medicine & Child Neurology*, 30, 502-508.

Aruin, A. S., & Almeida, G. L. (1997). A coactivation strategy in anticipatory postural adjustments in persons with Down syndrome. *Motor Control,* 1, 178-191.

Aruin, A. S., Shiratori, T., & Latash, M. L. (2001). The role of action in postural preparation for loading and unloading in standing subjects. *Experimental Brain Research,* 138, 458-466.

Assaiante, C. (1998). Development of locomotor balance control in healthy children. *Neuroscience Biobehavioral Review,* 22, 527-532.

Assaiante, C., Woollacott, M., & Amblard, B. (2000). Development of postural adjustment during gait initiation: Kinematic and EMG analysis. *Journal of Motor Behavior,* 32, 211-226.

Bai, D. L., Bertenthal, B. I. & Sussman, M. D. (1987). Children's sensitivity to optical flow for the control of stance. Abstracts of the third annual East Coast Clinical Gait Laboratory Conference. Bethesda, MD: National Institutes of Health.

Berger, W., Quintern, J. & Dietz, V. (1985). Stance and gait perturbations in children: Developmental aspects of compensatory mechanisms. *Electroencephalography & Clinical Neurophysiology,* 61, 385-395.

Bernstein, N. (1967). *Coordination and regulation of movements.* New York: NY: Pergamon.

Bertoti, D. B. (1986). Effect of short leg casting on ambulation in children with cerebral palsy. *Physical Therapy,* 66, 1522-1529.

Bertoti, D. B. (1988). Effect of therapeutic horseback riding on posture in children with cerebral palsy. *Physical Therapy,* 68, 1505-1511.

Bhattacharya, A., Shukla, R., Dietrich, K., Bornschein, R. & Berger, O. (1995). The effect of early lead exposure on children's postural balance. *Developmental Medicine and Child Neurology,* 37, 861-878.

Bjork, L., & Wetzel, A. (1983). A positional biofeedback device for sitting balance. *Physical Therapy,* 63, 1460-1461.

Boswell, B. (1991). Comparison of two methods of improving dynamic balance of mentally retarded children. *Perceptual & Motor Skills,* 73, 759-764.

Bouisset, S., Richardson, J., & Zattara, M. (2000). Are amplitude and duration of anticipatory postural adjustments identically scaled to focal movement parameters in humans? *Neuroscience Letters,* 278, 153-156.

Breniere, Y. & Bril, B. (1998). Development of postural control of gravity forces in children during the first 5 years of walking. *Experimental Brain Research,* 121, 3, 255-262.

Brogen, E., Forssberg, H. & Hadders-Algra, M. (2001). Influence of two different sitting positions on postural adjustments in children with spastic diplegia. *Developmental Medicine & Child Neurology,* 43, 534-546.

Brogen, E., Hadders-Algra, M. & Forssberg, H. (1998). Postural control in sitting children with cerebral palsy. *Neuroscience and Biobehavioral Reviews,* 22, 591-596.

Burleigh, A., & Horak, F. (1996). Influence of instruction, prediction, and afferent sensory information on the postural organization of step initiation. *Journal of Neurophysiology,* 75, 1619-1627.

Burleigh, A. L., Horak, F. B., & Malouin, F. (1994). Modification of postural responses and step initiation: Evidence for goal-directed postural interactions. *Journal of Neurophysiology,* 72, 2892-2902.

Burtner, P. A., Qualls, C., & Woollacott, M. H. (1998). Muscle activation characteristics of stance balance control in children with spastic cerebral palsy. *Gait and Posture,* 8, 163-174.

Burtner, P. A., Woollacott, M. H., & Qualls, C. (1999). Stance balance control with orthoses in a group of children with spastic cerebral palsy. *Developmental Medicine and Child Neurology,* 41, 748-757.

Butler, C., & Darrah, J. (2001) Effects of neurodevelopmental treatment (NDT) for cerebral palsy: An AACPDM evidence report. *Developmental Medicine and Child Neurology,* 43: 778-790.

Butler, P. B. (1998). A preliminary report of the effectiveness of trunk targeting in achieving independent sitting balance in children with cerebral palsy. *Clinical Rehabilitation,* 12, 281-293.

Butler, P. B., Thompson, N., & Major, R. E. (1992). Improvement in walking performance of children with cerebral palsy: Preliminary results. *Developmental Medicine & Child Neurology,* 34, 567-576.

Campbell, S. K. (1990). Effect of physical therapy in improving postural control in cerebral palsy. *Pediatric Physical Therapy,* 2, 135-140.

Carmick, J. (1993). Clinical use of neuromuscular electrical stimulation for children with cerebral palsy, Part 1: Lower extremity. *Physical Therapy,* 73, 505-513.

Carmick, J. (1995). Managing equinus in children with cerebral palsy: Electrical stimulation to strengthen the triceps surae muscle. *Developmental Medicine & Child Neurology,* 37, 965-975.

Casselbrandt, M. L., Redfern, M. S., Ferman, J. M., Fall, P. A. & Mandel, E. M. (1998). Visual-induced postural sway in children with otitis media. *Annuals of Otology, Rhinology and Laryngology,* 107, 401-405.

Chee, F. K. W., Kreutzberg, J. R., & Clark, D. L. (1978). Semicircular canal stimulation in cerebral palsied children. *Physical Therapy,* 58, 1071-1075.

Cherng, R. J., Chen, J. J., & Su, F. C. (2001). Vestibular system in performance of standing balance of children and young adults under altered sensory conditions. *Perceptual & Motor Skills,* 92, 1167-1179.

Corriveau, H., Hebert, R., Prince, F., & Raiche, M. (2000). Intrasession reliability of the "center of pressure minus center of mass" variable of postural control in the healthy elderly. *Archives of Physical Medicine & Rehabilitation,* 81, 45-48.

Daldeiden, S. (1990). Weight shifting as a treatment for balance deficits: A literature review. *Physiotherapy Canada,* 42, 81-87.

Damiano, D. L., Vaughan, C. L., & Abel, M. F. (1995). Muscle response to heavy resistance exercise in children with spastic cerebral palsy. *Developmental Medicine & Child Neurology,* 37, 731-739.

Damiano, D. L., Kelly, L. E., & Vaughn, C. L. (1995). Effects of quadriceps femoris muscle strengthening on crouch gait in children with spastic diplegia. *Physical Therapy,* 75, 658-667.

Deitz, J., Richardson, P. K., Westcott, S. L., & Crowe, T. K. (1996). Performance of children with learning disabilities on the Pediatric Clinical Test of Sensory Interaction for Balance. *Physical & Occupational Therapy in Pediatrics,* 16, 1-21.

Effgen, S. K. (1981) Effect of an exercise program on the static balance of deaf children. *Physical Therapy,* 61, 873-877.

Embrey, D.G., Yates, L., & Mott, D. (1990). Effects of neuro-developmental treatment and orthoses on knee flexion during gait: A single-subject design. *Physical Therapy, 70*, 626-637.

Ferdjallah, M., Harris, G. F., Smith, P. & Wertsch, J. J. (2002). Analysis of postural control synergies during quiet standing in healthy children and children with cerebral palsy. *Clinical Biomechanics, 17*, 203-210.

Fisher, A. G., & Bundy, A. C. (1982). Equilibrium reactions in normal children and in boys with sensory integrative dysfunctions. *Occupational Therapy Journal of Research, 2*, 171-183.

Forssberg, H. & Nashner, L. M. (1982). Ontogenic development of postural control in man: Adaptation to altered support and vision in man. *Journal of Neuroscience, 2*, 545-522.

Foster, E. C., Sveistrup, H. & Woollacott, M. H. (1996). Transitions in visual proprioception: Study of the effect of visual flow on postural control. *Journal of Motor Behavior, 28*, 101-112.

Frank, J. S. & Earl, M. (1990). Coordination of posture and movement. *Physical Therapy, 70*, 855-863.

Gabert, T. E., Jee, A., & Collins, W. E. (1982). Influence of passive and active vestibular stimulation on balance of young children. *Perceptual & Motor Skills, 54*, 548-550.

Gill, J., Allum, J. H., Carpenter, M. G., Held-Ziolkowska, M., Adkin, A. L., Honegger, F., & Pierchala, K. (2001). Trunk sway measures of postural stability during clinical balance tests: Effects of age. *Journal of Gerontology, 56*, M438-447.

Girolami, G. L., & Campbell, S. K. (1994). Efficacy of a neuro-developmental treatment program to improve motor control in infants born prematurely. *Pediatric Physical Therapy, 6*, 175-184.

Haas, G., Deiner, H. C., Rapp, H., & Dichgans, J. (1989). Development of feedback and feedforward control of upright stance. *Developmental Medicine & Child Neurology, 31*, 481-488.

Hadders-Algra, M., Brogren, E. & Forssberg, H. (1996a). Ontogeny of postural adjustments during sitting in infancy: Variation, selection and modulation. *Journal of Physiology, 493*, 273-288.

Hadders-Algra, M., Brogren, E. & Forssberg, H. (1996b). Training affects the development of postural adjustments in sitting infants. *Journal of Physiology, 493*, 289-298.

Hadders-Algra, M., Brogren, E. & Forssberg, H. (1997). Nature and nurture in the development of postural control in human infants. *Acta Paediatrics Supplement, 422*, 48-53.

Hadders-Algra, M., Brogren, E., & Forssberg, H. (1998). Postural adjustments during sitting at preschool age: Presence of a transient toddling phase. *Developmental Medicine Child Neurology, 40*, 436-447.

Hadders-Algra, M., van der Fits, I. B. M., Stremmelaar, E. F., & Touwen, B. C. L. (1999). Development of postural adjustments during reaching in infants with CP. *Developmental Medicine & Child Neurology, 41*, 766-776.

Harris, S. R., & Riffle, K. (1986). Effects of inhibitive ankle-foot orthoses on standing balance in a child with cerebral palsy. *Physical Therapy, 66*, 663-666.

Hartveld, A., & Hegarty, J. (1996). Frequent weightshift practice with computerized feedback by cerebral palsied children–four single-case experiments. *Physiotherapy, 82,* 573-580.

Hay, L., & Redon, C. (1999). Feedforward versus feedback control in children and adults subjected to a postural disturbance. *Experimental Brain Research, 125,* 153-162.

Hay, L., & Redon, C. (2001). Development of postural adaptations to arm raising. *Experimental Brain Research, 139,* 224-232.

Hinderer, K. A., Harris, S. H., Purdy, A., Chew D. E., Staheli, L. T., McLauglin, J.F., & Jaffe, K. M. (1988). Effects of "tone-reducing" vs. standard plaster-casts on gait improvement of children with cerebral palsy. *Developmental Medicine & Child Neurology, 30,* 370-377.

Hirschfeld, H., & Forssberg, H. (1991). Development of anticipatory postural adjustments during locomotion in children. *Journal of Neurophysiology, 66,* 12-19.

Hirschfeld, H., & Forssberg, H. (1992). Phase-dependent modulations of anticipatory postural adjustments during locomotion in children. *Journal of Neurophysiology, 68,* 542-550.

Hirschfeld, H. (1992). *On the integration of posture, locomotion, and voluntary movements in man: Normal and impaired development.* Stockholm: Nobel Institute of Neurophysics: Karolinksa Institute (Dissertation).

Hirschfeld, H. & Forssberg, H. (1994). Epigenetic development of postural responses for sitting during infancy. *Experimental Brain Research, 97,* 528-540.

Hopkins, B., & Ronnqvist, L. (2002). Facilitating postural control: Effects on the reaching behavior of 6-month-old infants. *Developmental Psychobiology, 40,* 168-182.

Horak, F. B. (1992). Motor control models underlying neurologic rehabilitation of posture in children. In: H. Forssberg, H. Hirschfeld (Eds.), Movement Disorders in Children. *Medicine & Sport Science,* Basel, Karger, 36, 21-30.

Horak, F. B., Shumway-Cook, A. & Black, F. O. (1988). Are vestibular deficits responsible for developmental disorders in children? *Insights in Otolaryngology* 3, 2-6.

Horak, F. B., Shumway-Cook, A., Crowe, T. K. & Black, F. O. (1988). Vestibular function and motor proficiency in children with hearing impairments and in learning disabled children with motor impairments. *Developmental Medicine and Child Neurology, 30, 64-79.*

Horvat, M. A. (1982). Effect of a home learning program on learning disabled children's balance. *Perceptual & Motor Skills, 55,* 1158.

Hulme, J. B., Shaver, J., Acher, S., Mullette, L., & Eggert, C. (1987). Effects of adaptive seating devices on the eating and drinking of children with multiple handicaps. *American Journal of Occupational Therapy, 41,* 81-89.

Jensen, J. & Bothner, K. (in press). Revisiting infant motor development schedules. The biomechanics of change. In: van Praagh (Ed.) *Anaerobic performance during childhood and adolescence.* Champaign, IL: Human Kinetics.

Jouen, F. (1984). Visual-vestibular interactions in infancy. *Infant Behavior and Development, 7,* 135-145.

Jouen, F. (1988). Visual-proprioceptive control of posture in newborn infants. In B. Amblard, A. Berthoz, F. Clarac (Eds.), *Posture and Gait: Development, Adaptation, and Modulation* (pp. 13-22). Amsterdam: Elsevier.

Jouen, F. (1993). Titres et travaux en vue de l'habilitation a diriger des recherches. State doctoral thesis. Paris: Universite Paris IV, 104.

Jouen, F. (in press). Early visual and vestibular relations in newborns. *Child Development.*

Kaminski, T. R., & Simpkins, S. (2001). The effects of stance configuration and target distance on reaching. I. Movement preparation. *Experimental Brain Research.* 136, 439-446.

Katic, R., Bonacin, D., & Blazevic, S. (2001). Phylogenetically conditioned possibilities of the realization and the development of complex movements at the age of 7 years. *Collegium Antropologicum,* 25, 573-583.

Kembhavi, G., Darrah, J., Magill-Evans, J., & Loomis, J. (2002). Using the Berg Balance Scale to distinguish balance abilities in children with cerebral palsy. *Pediatric Physical Therapy,* 14, 92-99.

Kokubun, M., Shinmyo, T., Ogita, M., Morita, K., Furuta, M., Haishi, K., Okuzumi, H., & Koike, T. (1997). Comparison of postural control on children with Down syndrome and those with other forms of mental retardation. *Perceptual & Motor Skills,* 84, 499-504.

Kuczynski, M., & Slonka, K. (1999). Influence of artificial saddle riding on postural stability in children with cerebral palsy. *Gait & Posture,* 10, 154-160.

Ledebt, A., Blandine, B., & Breniere, Y. (1998). The build-up of anticipatory behavior. *Experimental Brain Research,* 120, 9-17.

Lee, D., & Aronson, E. (1974). Visual proprioception control of standing in human infants. *Perception and Psychophysics,* 15, 529-532.

Le Pellec, A., & Maton, B. (1999). Anticipatory postural adjustments are associated with single vertical jump and their timing is predictive of jump amplitude. *Experimental Brain Research,* 129, 551-558.

Le Pellec, A., & Maton, B. (2000). Anticipatory postural adjustments depend on final equilibrium and task complexity in vertical jump movements. *Journal of Electromyography and Kinesiology,* 10, 171-178.

Le Pellec, A., & Maton, B. (2002). Initiation of a vertical jump: The human body's upward propulsion depends on control of forward equilibrium. *Neuroscience Letters,* 323, 183-186.

Lewis, S., Higham, L., & Cherry, D. (1985). Development of an exercise program to improve static and dynamic balance of profoundly hearing-impaired children. *American Annals of Deaf,* 130, 278-284.

Liao, H. F., Jeng, S. F., Lai, J. S., Cheng, C. K. & Hu, M. H. (1997). The relation between standing balance and walking function in children with spastic diplegia. *Developmental Medicine and Child Neurology,* 39, 106-112.

Lin, J. P., Brown, J. K., & Walsh, E. G. (1994). Physiological maturation of muscles in childhood. *Lancet,* 343, 1386-1389.

Liu, W. Y. (2001). *Anticipatory postural adjustments in children with cerebral palsy and children with typical development during forward reach tasks in standing.* Philadelphia, PA, MCP Hahnemann University (Dissertation, pp. 111-173).

Liu, W. Y., Zaino, C. A., & Westcott, S. L. (2000). Anticipatory postural adjustments in children with cerebral palsy and children with typical development during functional reaching: A center of pressure (COP) study. *Pediatric Physical Therapy,* 12, 218-219.

Lowes, L. P. (1997). *Evaluation of the standing balance of children with cerebral palsy and the tools for assessment.* Philadelphia, PA: Allegheny University of the Health Sciences (Dissertation).

MacPhail, A., Edwards, H. E., Golding, J., Miller, J., Carolyn, M., & Zwiers, T. (1998). Trunk posture reactions in children with and without cerebral palsy during therapeutic horseback riding. *Pediatric Physical Therapy,* 10, 143-147.

Malouin, F., & Richards, C. L. (2000). Preparatory adjustments during gait initiation in 4-6-year-old children. *Gait & Posture,* 11, 239-253.

Massion, J. (1992). Movement, posture and equilibrium: Interaction and coordination. *Progress in Neurobiology,* 38, 35-56.

Massion, J. (1994). Postural control system. *Current Opinion in Neurobiology,* 4, 877-887.

Mattiello, D., & Woollacott, M. (1997). Postural control in children: Development in typical populations and children with cerebral palsy and Down syndrome. In K. Connolly, H. Forssberg (Eds.), *Neurophysiology & Neuropsychology of Motor Development* (pp. 54-77). London, England: MacKeith Press.

McCollum, G. & Leen, T. K. (1989). Form exploration of mechanical stability limits in erect posture. *Journal of Motor Behavior,* 21, 225-244.

McGibbon, N. H., Andrade, C. K., Widener, G., & Cintas, H. L. (1998). Effect of an equine-movement therapy program on gait, energy expenditure, and motor function in children with spastic cerebral palsy: A pilot study. *Developmental Medicine & Child Neurology,* 40, 754-762.

Mesure, S., Amblard, B., & Cremieux, J. (1997). Effect of physical training on head-hip co-ordinated movements during unperturbed stance. *Neuroreport,* 8, 3507-3512.

Nashner, L. M. (1976). Adapting reflexes controlling the human posture. *Experimental Brain Research,* 26, 59-72.

Nashner, L. M. (1982). Adaptation of human movement to altered environments. *Trends in Neuroscience,* 358-361.

Nashner, L. M., Shumway-Cook, A. & Marin, O. (1983). Stance posture control in a select group of children with cerebral palsy: Deficits in sensory organization and motor coordination. *Experimental Brain Research,* 49, 393-409.

Norrlin, S., Karlsson, A., Ahlsten, G., Lanshammar, H., Silander, H. C., & Dahl, M. (2002). Force measurements of postural sway and rapid arm lift in seated children with and without MMC. *Clinical Biomechanics,* 17, 197-202.

Olney, S. J., & Wright, M. J. (2000). Cerebral palsy. In S.K. Campbell (Ed.), *Physical therapy for children* (pp. 533-570). Philadelphia, PA: WB Saunders.

Orner, C. E., Turner, D., & Worrell, T. (1994). Effect of foot orthoses on the balance skills of a child with a learning disability. *Pediatric Physical Therapy,* 6, 10-13.

Palisano, R., Rosenbaum, P., Walter, S., Russell, D., Wood, E., & Galuppi, B. (1997). Development and reliability of a system to classify gross motor function in children with cerebral palsy. *Developmental Medicine & Child Neurology,* 39, 214-223.

Philips, E. (2002). *Effect of a muscle strengthening program on spasticity, balance and functional skills in children with spasticity.* Albuquerque, NM: University of New Mexico. (Thesis).

Prechtl, H. F. R. (1997). The importance of fetal movements. In: K. J. Connolly & H. Forssberg (Eds.), *Neurophysiology and neuropsychology of motor development* (pp. 42-35). London, England: MacKeith Press.

Prechtl, H. F., & Hopkins, B. (1986). Developmental transformations of spontaneous movements in early infancy. *Early Human Development,* 14, 233-238.

Radtka, S. A., Skinner, S. R., Dixon, D. M., & Johanson, M. E. (1997). A comparison of gait with solid, dynamic, and no ankle-foot orthoses in children with spastic cerebral palsy. *Physical Therapy,* 77, 395-409.

Reid, D. T. (1996). The effects of the saddle seat on seated postural control and upper-extremity movement in children with cerebral palsy. *Developmental Medicine & Child Neurology,* 38, 805-815.

Rethlefsen, S., Kay, R., Dennis, S., Forstein, M., & Tolo, V. (1999). The effects of fixed and articulated ankle-foot orthoses on gait patterns in subjects with cerebral palsy. *Journal of Pediatric Orthopedics,* 19, 470-474.

Riach, C. L., & Hayes, K. C. (1989). Maturation of postural sway in young children. *Developmental Medicine & Child Neurology,* 29, 650-658.

Rine, R. M., Spielholtz, N., & Braswell, J. (2002). Emergence of alternate synergy in children with vestibular deficiency since birth. *Neuroscience Abstracts CD-ROM,* Program No. 666.16.

Roebuck, T. M.. Simmons, R. W., Richardson, C., Mattson, S. N. & Riley, E. P. (1998). Neuromuscular responses to disturbance in balance in children with prenatal exposure to alcohol. *Alcoholism, Clinical Experimental Research,* 22, 1992-1997.

Roncesvalles, N. C., & Jensen, J. (1993). The expression of weight bearing abilities in infants between four and seven months of age. *Sport and Exercise Psychology,* 15, 568.

Roncesvalles, N. C., Woollacott, M. H., & Jensen, J. L. (2000). Development of compensatory stepping skills in children. *Journal of Motor Behavior,* 32, 100-111.

Roncesvalles, N. C., Woollacott, M. H., & Jensen, J. L. (2001) Development of lower extremity kinetics for balance control in infants and young children. *Journal of Motor Behavior,* 33, 180-192.

Rose, J., Wolff, D. R., Jones, V. K., Bloch, D. A., Oehlert, J. W. & Gamble, J. G. (2002). Postural balance in children with cerebral palsy. *Developmental Medicine and Child Neurology 44,* 58-63.

Scherzer, A. L. & Tschamuter, I. (1990). *Early diagnosis and therapy in cerebral palsy: A primer on infant developmental problems.* (2nd ed.) New York, NY: Marcel Dekker.

Schloon, H., O'Brien, M. J., Scholten, C. A., & Prechtl, H. F. R. (1976). Muscle activity and postural behavior in newborn infants: A polymyographic study. *Neuropadiatrie,* 7, 384-415.

Schlosser, A., Philips, E., & Burtner, P. A. (2002). Effects of a muscle strengthening program on balance and function in children with spasticity. *Annual meeting of the American Occupational Therapy Association.* Orlando, FL.

Schmidt, R.A. (1988). *Motor Control and Learning* (2nd ed.). Champaign, IL: Human Kinetics.

Schmitz, C., Martin, N., & Assaiante, C. (1999). Development of anticipatory postural adjustments in a bimanual load-lifting task in children. *Experimental Brain Research*, 126, 200-204.

Selz, P. A., Girardi, M., Konrad, H. R., & Hughes, L. F. (1996). Vestibular deficits in deaf children. *Otolaryngology Head and Neck Surgery*, 115, 70-77.

Shepherd, R. B. (1995). *Physiotherapy in paediatrics*. Oxford, England: Butterworth-Heinemann.

Shiratori, T., & Latash, M. (2000). The roles of proximal and distal muscles in anticipatory postural adjustments under asymmetrical perturbations and during standing on rollerskates. *Clinical Neurophysiology*, 111, 613-623.

Shiratori, T., & Latash, M. (2001). Anticipatory postural adjustments during load catching by standing subjects. *Clinical Neurophysiology*, 112, 1250-1265.

Shumway-Cook, A., & McCollum, G. (1991). Assessment and treatment of balance deficits. In P. C. Montgomery, B. H. Connolly (Eds). *Motor Control and Physical Therapy Theoretical Framework and Practical Applications* (pp. 123-137). Hixson, TN: Chattanooga Group Inc.

Shumway-Cook, A. & Woollacott, M. (1985a). The growth of stability: Postural control from a developmental perspective. *Journal of Motor Behavior*, 17, 131-147.

Shumway-Cook, A. & Woollacott, M.H. (1985b). Postural control in the Down's Syndrome child. *Physical Therapy*, 9, 161-171.

Shumway-Cook, A. & Woollacott, M. (1993). Theoretical issues in assessing postural control. In I. J. Wilhelm (Ed.) *Clinics in physical therapy: Physical therapy assessment in infancy* (pp. 161-171). New York, NY: Churchill Livingstone.

Shumway-Cook, A. & Woollacott, M. H. (2001). *Motor Control: Theory and Practical Applications (2nd Ed.)*. Baltimore, MD: Lippincott, Wilkins & Williams.

Shumway-Cook, A., Woollacott, M. H., Hutchinson, S., Kartin, D. & Price, R. (submitted). The effect of balance training on recovery of stability in children with cerebral palsy. *Developmental Medicine and Child Neurology*.

Slijper, H., & Latash, M. (2000). The effects of instability and additional land support on anticipatory postural adjustments in leg, trunk, and arm muscles during standing. *Experimental Brain Research*, 135, 81-93.

Slijper, H., Latash, M. L., & Mordkoff, J. T. (2002). Anticipatory postural adjustments under simple and choice reaction time conditions. *Brain Research*, 924, 184-197.

Smyth, N.M., & Mason, U. C. (1998). Use of proprioception in normal and clumsy children. *Developmental Medicine and Child Neurology*, 40, 672-681.

Sundermier, L. & Woollacott, M. H. (1998). The influence of vision on the automatic postural muscle responses in newly standing and newly walking infants. *Experimental Brain Research*, 120, 537-540.

Sundermier, L., Woollacott, M. H., Roncevalles, R. C., & Jensen, J. L. (2001). The development of balance control in children: Comparisons of EMG and kinetic variables and chronological and developmental groupings. *Experimental Brain Research*, 136, 340-350.

Sveistrup, H., & Woollacott, M. H. (1996). Longitudinal development of the automatic postural response in infants. *Journal of Motor Behavior*, 28, 58-70.

Sveistrup, H., & Woollacott, M. H. (1997). Practice modifies the developing automatic postural response. *Experimental Brain Research*, 114, 33-43.

Sveistrup, H., & Woollacott, M. H., Shumway-Cook, A., & McCollum, G. (1990). A longitudinal study on the transition to independent stance in children. *Neuroscience Abstracts,* 16, 893.

Tardieu, G., Tardieu, C., Colbeau-Justin, P., & Lespargot, A. (1982). Muscle hypoextensibility in children with cerebral palsy: II Therapeutic implications. *Archives of Physical Medicine & Rehabilitation,* 63, 103-107.

Thelen, E. (1986). Development of coordinated movement: Implications for early human development. In M. G. Wade & H. T. A. Whiting (Eds.). *Motor development in children: Aspects of coordination and control* (pp. 107-124). Dordect, the Netherlands: Martinus Nijhoff Publishers.

Thelen, E., & Spencer, J. P. (1998). Postural control during reaching in young infants: A dynamic systems approach. *Neuroscience and Biobehavioral Reviews,* 22, 507-514.

Thorpe, D. E., & Valvano, J. (2002). The effects of knowledge of performance and cognitive strategies on motor skill learning in children with cerebral palsy. *Pediatric Physical Therapy,* 14, 2-15.

Thorpe, D., Zaino, C., Westcott, S., & Valvano, J. (1998). Comparison of postural muscle coordination patterns during a functional reaching task in typically developing children and children with cerebral palsy. *Physical Therapy,* 78, S80-81.

Van der Fits, I. B. M., Hadders-Algra, M. (1998). The development of postural response patterns during reaching in healthy infants. *Neuroscience and Biobehavioral Reviews,* 22, 521-526.

Van der Fits, I. B., Klip, A. W., van Eykern, L. A., & Hadders-Algra, M. (1999). Postural adjustments during spontaneous and goal-directed arm movements in the first half year of life. *Behavioral Brain Research,* 106, 75-90.

Van der Fits, I. B., Otten, E., Klip, A. W., Van Eykern, L. A., & Hadders-Algra, M. (1999). The development of postural adjustments during reaching in 6- to 18-month-old infants: Evidence for two transitions. *Experimental Brain Research,* 126, 517-528.

Vereijken, B., van Emmerick, R. E. A., Whiting, H. T. A., & Newell, K. M. (1992). Free(z)ing degrees of freedom in skill acquisition. *Journal of Motor Behavior,* 24, 133-142.

Wang, W. Y., & Chang, J. J. (1997). Effects of jumping skill training on walking balance for children with mental retardation and Down syndrome. *Kaohsiung Journal of Medical Science,* 13, 487-495.

Watt, J., Sims, D., Harckham, F., Schmidt, L., McMillan, A., & Hamilton, J. (1986). A prospective study of inhibitive casting as an adjunct to physiotherapy for cerebral palsied children. *Developmental Medicine & Child Neurology,* 28, 480-488.

Westcott, S. L. (2001). Examination/Evaluation and Interventions for Children with Postural Control Disorders. (Lesson 7) In APTA Topics in Physical Therapy: Pediatrics Home Study Course (pp. 1-35). Alexandria, VA: American Physical Therapy Association.

Westcott, S. L., Hartzler-Murray, K., & Pence, K. (1998). Survey of preferences of pediatric physical therapists for assessment and treatment of balance dysfunction in children. *Pediatric Physical Therapy,* 10, 48-61.

Westcott, S. L., & Lowes, L. P. (1995). Commentary on: Effects of quadriceps femoris muscle strengthening on crouch gait in children with spastic diplegia. *Physical Therapy,* 75, 668-669.

Westcott, S. L., Lowes, L. P., Richardson, P. K., Crowe, T. K., & Deitz, J. (1997). Difference in the use of sensory information for maintenance of standing balance in children with different motor disabilities. *Developmental Medicine & Child Neurology,* 39 (Suppl 75), 32-33.

Westcott, S. L., Richardson, P. K., & Lowes, L. P. (1997). Evaluation of postural stability in children: Current theories and assessment tools. *Physical Therapy,* 77, 629-645.

Westcott, S. L., & Zaino, C. A. (1997). Comparison and development of postural muscle activity in children during stand and reach from firm and compliant surfaces. *Society for Neuroscience Abstracts,* 23, 1565.

Westcott, S. L., Zaino, C. A., Miller, F., & Thorpe, D. E. (1997). Comparison of postural muscle activity in children of different ages during stand and reach from firm, compliant, and narrow surfaces. *Pediatric Physical Therapy,* 9, 207.

Westcott, S. L., Zaino, C. A., Miller, F., Thorpe, D., & Unanue, R. (1998). Anticipatory postural coordination and functional movement skills by degree of cerebral palsy in children age 6-12 years. *Society for Neuroscience Abstracts,* 24, 149.

Westcott, S. L., Zaino, C. A., Unanue, R., Thorpe, D., & Miller, F. (1998). Comparison of anticipatory postural control and dynamic balance ability in children with and without cerebral palsy. *Developmental Medicine & Child Neurology,* 40(Suppl 78), 14.

Wiley, M. E., & Damiano, D. L. (1998). Lower-extremity strength profiles in spastic cerebral palsy. *Developmental Medicine & Child Neurology,* 40, 100-107.

Winstein, C. J. (1991). Designing practice for motor learning: Clinical implications. In: M. J. Lister (Ed.) *Contemporary management of motor problems: Proceedings of the II Step Conference* (pp. 65-76). Alexandria,VA: American Physical Therapy Association.

Winstein, C. J., Gardner, E. R., McNeal, D. R., Barto, P. S., & Nicholson, D. E. (1989). Standing balance training: Effect on balance and locomotion in hemiparetic adults. *Archives of Physical Medicine & Rehabilitation,* 70, 755-762.

Winter, D. (1990). *Biomechanics and motor control of human movement.* New York, NY: John Wiley and Sons.

Witherington, D. C., von Hofsten, C., Rosander, K., Robinette, A., Woollacott, M.H., & Bertenthal, B. I. (2002). The development of anticipatory postural adjustments in infancy. *Infancy,* 3, 495-517.

Woollacott, M. H., Burtner, P., Jensen, J., Jasiewicz, J., Roncesvalles, N., & Sveistrup, H. (1998). Development of postural responses during standing in healthy children and children with spastic diplegia. *Neuroscience & Biobehavioral Reviews,* 22, 583-589.

Woollacott, M., Debu, B., & Mowatt, M. (1987). Neuromuscular posture of the infant and child: Is vision dominant? *Journal of Motor Behavior,* 19, 167-186.

Woollacott, M. H., & Jensen, J. L. (1996). Posture and gait. In H. Heuer & S. Keele (Eds). *Handbook of perception and action, Vol. 2* (pp. 333-403). San Diego, CA: Academic Press.

Woollacott, M. H., & Shumway-Cook, A. (1986). The development of postural and voluntary motor control systems in Down Syndrome children. In M. G. Wade (Ed.) *Motor skill acquisition in the mentally handicapped: Issues in research and training* (pp. 45-71). Amsterdam, Holland: Elsevier.

Woollacott, M. H., & Shumway-Cook, A. (1994). Maturation of feedback control of posture and equilibrium. In E. Fedrizzi, G. Avanzini, & P. Crenna (Eds.) *Motor development in children* (pp. 59-70). London, England: John Libbey & Co.

Woollacott, M. H., Shumway-Cook, A., & Williams, H. G. (1989). The development of posture and balance control in children. In M. H. Woollacott, & A. Shumway-Cook (Eds). *Development of posture and gait across the life span* (pp. 77-96). Columbia, SC: University of South Carolina Press.

Woollacott, M. H. & Sveistrup, H. (1992). Changes in the sequencing and timing of muscle coordination associated with developmental transitions in balance abilities. *Human Movement Science, 11*, 23-36.

Woollacott, M. H., von Hosten, C., & Rosblad, B. (1998). Relation between muscle responses onset and body segmental movements during postural perturbations in humans. *Experimental Brain Research, 72*, 593-604.

Zaino, C. A. (1999). *Motor control of a functional reaching task in children with cerebral palsy and children with typical development: A comparison of electromyographic and kinetic measurements.* Philadelphia, PA: Allegheny University of the Health Sciences (Dissertation, pp. 50-104).

Zaino, C. A., & Westcott, S. L. (1997). Comparison of postural muscle activity patterns during a functional reaching task in typically developing children and children with cerebral palsy. *Society for Neuroscience Abstracts, 23*, 2375.

Zaino, C. A., Westcott, S. L., Ideishi, R. I., & Gocha, V. (1999). Comparison of electromyographical and kinetic measures of postural control during weighted and non-weighted reaches in children with typical development. *Pediatric Physical Therapy, 11*, 224.

Zaino, C. A., Westcott, S. L., Miller, F., & Thorpe, D. E. (1998). Comparison of postural muscle motor coordination patterns and learning effects in children who are typically developing and children who have cerebral palsy while on compliant and non-compliant surfaces. *Pediatric Physical Therapy, 10*, 71.

Zimmerman, A. W., Gross, K. C., & Speckhart, F. H. (1993). Vestibular stimulation: A device for off-vertical axis rotation. *Infants & Young Children, 6*, 56-67.

Muscle Force and Range of Motion as Predictors of Standing Balance in Children with Cerebral Palsy

Linda Pax Lowes
Sarah L. Westcott
Robert J. Palisano
Susan K. Effgen
Margo N. Orlin

SUMMARY. Children with cerebral palsy frequently receive therapeutic intervention to remediate standing balance deficits. Evaluation of the impairments associated with poor balance could facilitate more effective treatment programs. This study evaluated the relationship between

Linda Pax Lowes, PT, PhD, PCS, is Adjunct Faculty, Department of Physical Therapy, The Ohio State University, and Physical Therapist at Getting Started, Columbus, Ohio. Sarah L. Westcott, PT, PhD, is Adjunct Associate Professor, Drexel University, Philadelphia, PA, and Physical Therapist at the Lake Washington School District, Redmond, WA. Robert J. Palisano, PT, ScD, is Professor, Programs in Rehabilitation Sciences, Drexel University. Susan K. Effgen, PT, PhD, holds a Joseph Hamburg Professorship in Rehabilitation Sciences, and is Director, Rehabilitation Sciences Doctoral Program, College of Health Sciences, University of Kentucky. Margo N. Orlin, PT, MS, PCS, is Assistant Professor, Programs in Rehabilitation Sciences, Drexel University.

Address correspondence to: Linda Pax Lowes, PT, PhD, PCS, 2221 North Star Road, Columbus, OH 43221 (E-mail: lpax@yahoo.com).

[Haworth co-indexing entry note]: "Muscle Force and Range of Motion as Predictors of Standing Balance in Children with Cerebral Palsy." Lowes et al. Co-published simultaneously in *Physical & Occupational Therapy in Pediatrics* (The Haworth Press, Inc.) Vol. 24, No. 1/2, 2004, pp. 57-77; and: *Movement Sciences: Transfer of Knowledge into Pediatric Therapy Practice* (ed: Robert J. Palisano) The Haworth Press, Inc., 2004, pp. 57-77. Single or multiple copies of this article are available for a fee from The Haworth Document Delivery Service [1-800-HAWORTH, 9:00 a.m. - 5:00 p.m. (EST). E-mail address: docdelivery@haworthpress.com].

lower extremity force production, range of motion and standing balance in thirty-five children between the ages of 6 and 14 years of age with spastic cerebral palsy. Standing balance was evaluated using the Pediatric Clinical Test of Sensory Interaction (P-CTSIB). Hand-held dynamometry was used to assess force production and goniometry was used to assess range of motion. The results indicated that force production and range of motion are highly related to standing balance. Blocked, hierarchical multiple regression analysis revealed that force production explained 41% of the variance in P-CTSIB scores in this sample, while range of motion explained an additional 13%. Therefore, the total variance explained by these variables was 54%. Results of this study suggest that impairment level testing may allow the development of more effective individualized intervention programs to remediate balance deficits. Clinical suggestions are provided. *[Article copies available for a fee from The Haworth Document Delivery Service: 1-800-HAWORTH. E-mail address: <docdelivery@ haworthpress.com> Website: <http://www.HaworthPress.com> © 2004 by The Haworth Press, Inc. All rights reserved.]*

KEYWORDS. Cerebral palsy, balance, range of motion, strength, children

Promoting balance in standing during daily activities and routines is an outcome of therapy intervention for children with cerebral palsy (CP) (Horak & Shumway-Cook, 1990; Palisano et al., 1997; Shumway- Cook & Woollacott, 2001). Children with CP have been documented to have poorer balance abilities in standing compared to typically developing peers (Thorpe & Westcott, 1998; Woollacott, Burtner, & Jensen, 1998). Based on models of disablement, balance disorders can be examined on many levels (World Health Organization, 2001). Therapists frequently evaluate the impact balance has on the child's ability to perform functional skills such as walking and dressing. Balance can also be evaluated independent of functional task through perturbations, on tilt boards, or through weight shifting. Knowledge of the neuromuscular and musculoskeletal impairments that interact with the standing balance of children with CP would have application to physical and occupational therapy examination, prognosis, and intervention.

Systems theory of motor control provides a framework for inquiry into how neuromuscular and musculoskeletal impairments influence standing balance. In systems theory, the nervous system is conceptualized as part of a flexible complex of systems and subsystems that control movement (Shumway-Cook & Woollacott, 2001). Movement is viewed as an emergent property from the interaction of the neuromuscular system, musculoskeletal system, central nervous system, and features of the environment influencing the movement. Horak and Shumway-Cook (1986) developed the Sensory Organization Test to determine the influence of multiple sensory systems of the ability of adults to maintain balance. Based on this work, the Pediatric Clinical Test of Sensory Interactions for Balance (P-CTSIB) (Crowe, Deitz, Richardson, & Atwater, 1990; Deitz, Richardson, Atwater, Crowe, & Odiorne, 1991; Richardson, Atwater, Crowe, & Deitz, 1992; Westcott, Crowe, Deitz, & Richardson, 1994) was developed to assess children. By systematically manipulating the sensory input the child receives, the P-CTSIB evaluates the contributions of the child's visual, somatosensory (proprioceptive/cutaneous), and vestibular systems in maintaining standing balance.

Impaired *force production* is a component of the movement disorder in children with spastic CP (Damiano, Martellotta, Quinlivan, & Abel, 2001; Wiley & Damiano, 1998). Impairment in muscle force production is a multifactorial problem. Children with CP have abnormalities in muscle composition (Rose, Haskell, Gamble, Hamilton, Brown, & Rinsky, 1994) that may contribute to poor force production. Increased muscle stiffness and range of motion limitations can alter muscle length/tension curves, and may result in insufficient force output during movement. Impairments in the neuromuscular system limit the ability to coordinate muscle timing and force production to external conditions (Burtner, Qualls, & Woollacott, 1998; Burtner, Woollacott, & Qualls, 1999; Thorpe, Zaino, Westcott, & Valvano, 1998). Force production is important because it is related to efficiency of standing and walking (Damiano, Quinlivan, Owen, Shaffrey, & Abel, 2001; Damiano, Kelly & Vaughn, 1995; Kramer & MacPhail, 1994; Parker, Carriere, Hebestreit, Salsberg, & Bar-Or, 1993). Children with CP are able to increase force production with strength training without adverse effects such as increased spasticity (Dodd, Taylor, & Damiano, 2002). Damiano, Martellotta, Quinlivan, and Abel (2001) reported that force output gains followed a normal strengthening curve characterized by an initial rapid increase in strength attributable to motor learning followed by a slower rate of increase in strength attributable to muscle hypertrophy. The relationship between force output level and standing balance abilities, however, has not been determined.

Range of motion limitations can adversely affect standing balance in several ways. Knee flexion contractures have been shown to affect balance. Postural sway was increased in subjects with simulated knee flexion contractures of both 15 and 30 degrees (Potter, Kirby, & MacLeod, 1990). Knee contractures of this magnitude can be seen in children with cerebral palsy. Similarly, ankle range of motion limitations could interfere with balance by impeding the use of an ankle strategy for postural adjustments. A child's base of support is also influenced by range of motion. The common stance of children with diplegia; ankle plantarflexion, hip internal rotation and adduction, considerably narrows the child's base of support. A small base of support accentuates the impact of external perturbations, therefore challenging balance.

The purpose of this study was to examine the relationship between isometric muscle force, joint range of motion, and standing balance abilities in children with CP who are able to walk independently or with an assistive device [levels I, II and III on the Gross Motor Function Classification System (Palisano et al., 1997)]. We hypothesized that isometric muscle force and passive joint range of motion in the legs will explain a significant percentage of the variance in standing balance abilities of children with CP. Knowledge of the percentage of variance in standing balance abilities explained by isometric muscle force and passive joint range of motion has direct implications for procedural interventions to improve standing balance in children with CP.

METHODS

Subjects

Subjects were recruited through the A. I. duPont Institute Cerebral Palsy Clinic, Motion Analysis Laboratory and Physical Therapy Department. Subjects had a diagnosis of spastic CP and were between ages 6 through 14 years. The lower age of six years was selected because children younger than this age rely predominantly on visual information for balance reactions. After the age of six years, typically developing children incorporate sensory information from the visual, somatosensory and vestibular systems for balance (Forssberg & Nashner, 1982; Foudriat et al., 1993; Woollacott et al., 1989). Approval from the Hahnemann University Institutional Review Board and the Alfred I. duPont Institute was obtained.

Thirty-five subjects, 18 boys and 17 girls, between the ages of 6 years and 14 years (X = 10 years, SD = 2.7) participated in the study. Twenty-four of the subjects have spastic diplegic, eight have spastic hemiplegia, and three have spastic quadriplegia. Inclusion criteria were a diagnosis of spastic CP and the ability to stand independently for 30 seconds without orthotic devices. Exclusion criteria were as follows: use of a hearing aid, blindness, history of a dorsal rhizotomy surgery, history of an orthopedic surgery or fracture in the previous six months. There was not a statistically significant difference in the age of the children by gender (p = .10) or diagnosis (p = .68).

Tests and Measures

The measures were specifically chosen because they are feasible to administer in clinical practice.

The Pediatric Clinical Test of Sensory Interaction for Balance (P-CTSIB)

The Pediatric Clinical Test of Sensory Interactions for Balance (P-CTSIB) (Crowe et al., 1990; Deitz et al., 1991; Richardson et al., 1992; Westcott et al., 1994) was developed based on the work of Horak and Shumway-Cook (1986) who originally developed a clinical test to replicate the information obtained through computerized posturography using equipment assembled easily by a clinician. The P-CTSIB uses high-density foam to provide inaccurate somatosensory information and a visual conflict dome to provide inaccurate visual information. By systematically manipulating the sensory input the child receives, the P-CTSIB evaluates the contributions of the child's visual, somatosensory and vestibular systems in maintaining standing balance.

The P-CTSIB creates six different sensory conditions by using a firm or compliant surface, having the eyes open or closed, or wearing a visual conflict dome to systematically manipulate the sensory information available to the child for maintaining balance (see Figure 1).

Dietz et al. (1991) and Richardson et al. (1992) examined differences in P-CTSIB performance in children between the ages of four to nine years old. The four and five-year-old children had difficulty maintaining balance with eyes closed. Inter-rater reliability of the P-CTSIB is supported by Spearman rank order correlation coefficients of > .80 in four of the six conditions. The two exceptions were condition 3 (r = .69) and condition 4 (r = .79). The authors hypothesized that the lower reli-

FIGURE 1. The following order of testing was used throughout the study and is theorized to represent the order of increasing difficulty.

Condition 1: Eyes open / Firm surface
Condition 2: Eyes closed / Firm surface
Condition 3: Visual conflict dome /Firm surface
Condition 4: Eyes open / Foam surface
Condition 5: Eyes closed / Foam surface
Condition 6: Visual conflict dome / Foam surface

The criteria for scoring each condition are:
0 = Child cannot assume the position
1 = Child maintains stance 3 seconds or less
2 = Child maintains stance 4-10 seconds
3 = Child maintains stance 11-29 seconds, or 30 seconds with > 15 degrees of sway
4 = Child maintains stance 30 seconds with > 5 degrees but < 15 degrees of sway
5 = Child maintains stance 30 seconds with 5 degrees or less of sway

ability might have been attributable to a small range of obtained scores (Crowe et al., 1990). For test-retest reliability, Spearman coefficients range from .45 for the vision accurate category to .69 vision inaccurate (Westcott et al., 1994). In inter-rater reliability testing in children with developmental delays, interclass correlation coefficients ranged from 0.55-0.88 (ICC 2,1) (Pellegrino, Buelow, Krause, Loucks, & Westcott, 1995).

Hand-Held Dynamometry

Isometric muscle force production was measured using a Nicholas Manual Muscle Tester[1] (MMT) Model 01160 which is a small, light-weight, easy to read dynamometer that uses a digital display to record the peak force exerted during each trial. It has an accuracy of +/− 0.5 percent between 0.0 to 199.9 kilograms (440 pounds) (Lafayette Instrument). Dynamometry has been demonstrated to be a reliable measure of force output in a variety of clinical populations and in children as young as three years old (Dichter, 1994; Dvir, Bar-Haim, & Arvel, 1990; Effgen & Brown, 1992; Gajdosik, Nelson, & Gleason, 1994; Horvat, Croce, & Roswal, 1994; Hunt, 1995). Two valid measurements were taken and the higher value was used for data analysis.

Range of Motion

Measuring range of motion in individuals with spasticity can be problematic and unreliable (Harris, Harthun Smith, & Krukowski, 1985; Stuberg, Fuchs, & Miedaner, 1988). To ensure adequate reliability, a single examiner collected all the data following the guidelines of Norkin and White (1985). Passive range of motion was performed several times before the measurements were taken. The limb was moved slowly and sustained end pressure was applied while the measurement was taken. Two valid measures were taken for each joint and higher value was used for data analysis.

Reliability

The first author collected all the study data with the exception of the timing component of the P-CTSIB. Timing was completed by one of three experienced assistants. Prior to data collection, the ability of the first author to administer the measures reliably was determined with a group of children who were similar in age and/or abilities to the subjects. Reliability checks were also performed midway through data collection using study participants.

Prior to data collection, the first author and an experienced assistant established inter-rater reliability for the P-CTSIB on 14 children. The overall Kappa coefficient for time/sway categories was .88 and ranged from .60-1.00 for each condition, while percent agreement was 93% overall and ranged from 86-100%. Midway through the data collection, the first two authors independently scored the tests of 8 subjects. The overall Kappa coefficient was .84 and ranged from .67-1.0 for each condition. The percent agreement also remained high at 89% overall and ranged from 83-100% for each condition. For both trials, 100% of the scores were within one point of each other. All P-CTSIB study data was collected by the first author.

Inter-rater reliability of dynamometry was established prior to data collection by the first author and two experienced clinicians who each measured 5 (knee flexion) to 8 (hip flexion) muscle groups. Intra-class correlation coefficients (ICC) (3,1) ranged from .94 (hip flexion) to .99 (hip abduction, knee flexion, ankle dorsiflexion). Midway through data collection inter-reliability remained similarly high when tested on 7 (hip flexion) to 9 (ankle plantar and dorsiflexion) muscle groups, with ICCs (3,1) ranging from .96 (plantarflexion) to .99 (hip extension and abduction).

Inter-rater reliability of goniometric measurements was established by the first author and two experienced clinicians on a group of six children with CP. Intra-class correlation coefficients (3,1) ranged from .85 for ankle eversion to 1.00 for knee extension and ankle inversion. A reliability check was performed midway through data collection on four children who were participating in the study. Due to the small sample size and limited range in the data, the ICC values may be misleading.

Therefore, the data were evaluated as the degrees difference between the two raters over four trials. The largest difference for one trial was eight degrees and occurred once on foot inversion and once on knee flexion. The mean difference for the four limbs for each joint motion ranged from perfect agreement for knee extension to 4.5 degrees for foot inversion.

Procedures

Pediatric Test of Sensory Interaction for Balance

Equipment used to administer the P-CTSIB included a sway backdrop with degree of sway markings, visual conflict dome, medium density closed cell foam, and a stop watch. The visual conflict dome moves with the child's body and therefore gives the visual perception that the child is not swaying. The standing surface consists of either the level floor or an 18 × 16 inch piece of closed cell foam. The foam conforms to the weight of the child and provides decreased proprioceptive input and inaccurate cutaneous input from the ankle.

The child was instructed to stand up straight with feet together and hands on the hips. The feet were positioned so that both the malleoli and the first metatarsal heads were touching. If the child could not assume this position, the closest approximation was accepted. If the child was unable to assume the feet together position due to poor balance the child received a score of 0 for that trial. The amount of time the child remained standing, up to 30 seconds, was recorded for each test condition. The trial was stopped prior to thirty seconds if the child required assistance to keep from falling, took a step or moved their feet out of the testing position, removed their hands from their hips, or opened their eyes during one of the vision absent conditions. The amount of sway in both a forward and backward direction was also recorded. Each child was given two trials in each condition. The total degrees of sway and the number of seconds the child remained standing were used to assign the child's performance an ordinal score.

Muscle Isometric Force

The following muscle groups were tested bilaterally in the standard positions described by Bohannon (1986, 1987): hip flexion, extension and abduction, and ankle dorsiflexion and plantarflexion. Knee flexion and extension testing positions were modified from a sitting position to a prone position (Dichter, 1994) to eliminate the need to maintain sitting balance while performing a maximum voluntary contraction.

Prior to testing each muscle, the children performed both passive and active range of motion. When the child demonstrated the ability to activate the desired muscle by performing the concentric contraction, the child was asked to perform an isometric contraction of the muscle against the investigator's hand. The child was then instructed to push against the muscle tester in the specified direction as hard as they could for 4-5 seconds (Effgen & Brown, 1992). The child was given two trials. If there was a discrepancy of greater than 10% additional trials were administered until two valid trials within 10% of one another were obtained. None of the children required more than four trials.

Goniometry

Lower extremity ROM was measured bilaterally. Two measurements were taken at each joint. If there was a discrepancy of greater than 10% between the two measurements additional trials were administered until two valid trials within 10% of one another were obtained. None of the children required more than four trials.

Data Analysis

A data screening was performed to ascertain whether the data met the assumptions for parametric statistical analysis. Several of the variables were not normally distributed so logarithmic transformation was performed on these variables to allow for use of parametric statistics. All of the children completed all of the testing with the exception of knee flexion and extension where one child could not assume the testing position.

Data were analyzed using a theory generated blocked hierarchical multiple regression. The two blocks entered were force output and range of motion. Systems theory states that motor behavior is derived from the interaction of body components (Shumway-Cook & Woollacott, 2001). This would suggest that the sum of the available range and force capabilities is more important than any single variable. Theoretical rationale and correlation values were used to reduce the number of data in each of the two blocks (Tables 1 and 2).

The force output from the following muscle groups were entered together as the first block: hip extension, abduction, knee extension, ankle dorsiflexion and plantarflexion. Hip extension was entered because of

TABLE 1. Correlations Between Muscle Force (Kilograms) Measurements in Children with Cerebral Palsy

	Hip Flexion	Hip Extension	Hip Abduction	Knee Extension	Knee Flexion	Dorsiflexion
Hip Flexion		.44**	.81**	.19	.06	.80**
Hip Extension	.44**		.70**	.15	−.19	.86**
Hip Abduction	.81**	.70**		.19	−.04	.74**
Knee Extension	.19	.15	.19		.91**	.32
Knee Flexion	.06	−.19	−.04	.91**		.16
Dorsiflexion	.80**	.49**	.74**	.32	.16	
Plantarflexion	.68**	.67**	.74**	.14	−0.4	.66**

* p = .05 ** p = .01

TABLE 2. Correlations Between Passive Joint Range of Motion Measurements in Children with Cerebral Palsy

	H Flex	H Ext	H Abd	H ER	H IR	K Flex	K Ext	Dorsi	Plantar	Inver
Hip Flex		.04	.58**	.32	.30	.55**	−.21	.49**	.49**	.61**
Hip Ext	0.4		.12	−.13	.18	−.06	.34*	.24	.06	.27
Hip Abd	.58**	.12		.36*	.31	.45**	−.04	.31	.37*	.63**
Hip Ext Rot	.32	−.13	.36*		.18	.39*	−.11	−.05	.40*	.16
Hip Int Rot	.30	.18	.31	.18		.08	.17	.36	.07	.46**
Knee Flex	.55**	−.06	−.04	.39*	.08		−.10	.38*	.41*	.43*
Knee Ext	−.21	.34*	.45**	−.11	.17	−.10		−.17	.04	.18
Dorsiflex	.49**	.24	.31	−.05	.36*	.38*	−.17		−.14	.41*
Plantarflex	.49**	.06	.37*	.40*	.07	.41*	.04	−.14		.35*
Inversion	.61**	.27	.63**	.16	.46**	.43*	.18	.41*	.35*	
Eversion	.23	.14	.35*	.34*	.51	.37*	−.03	.42*	.13	.49**

*p = .05 ** p = .01

its importance in performing a hip strategy for maintaining balance. Abduction was entered because it provides stability in the saggital plane. Knee extension was entered because of its role in stabilizing the knee. Finally, both ankle plantarflexion and dorsiflexion were entered because of their role in performing an ankle strategy balance maneuver. Knee flexion was excluded because it was highly correlated to knee extension ($r = .91$, $p = .01$). In addition the testing position for knee flexion was at or near the end of the majority of the children's range of motion so 65% of the children were unable to generate sufficient force to register on the dynamometer. Similarly, hip flexion was excluded because

43% of the children were unable to generate sufficient force to register on the dynamometer.

The range of motion block was entered next and included: hip extension and external rotation, and ankle dorsiflexion and eversion. In the range of motion variables, none of the variables were intercorrelated above .61 (Table 2). In general, the range of motion lacking in the typical posture of the child with cerebral palsy was entered into the regression. Typical lower extremity standing posture for children with cerebral palsy is hip flexion, hip internal rotation and ankle planterflexion. Therefore ankle dorsiflexion, hip extension and hip external rotation were entered into the regression. The exception to this general rule was the inclusion of foot eversion. Overall, the children in this study showed excessive foot eversion. Excessive eversion could be an indication of a collapsed longitudinal arch and could indicate foot instability that would have a negative impact on the child's P-CTSIB scores. Abduction was not entered because overall, this was not an area of limitation for the children and the testing position for the P-CTSIB is with the feet together, therefore abduction range was not required. Both knee flexion and extension were excluded. Knee flexion was eliminated because a person needs little if any motion in this direction to maintain quiet standing. Knee extension was not included because both limitations and excesses were seen in this sample of children with CP. It was hypothesized that both abnormalities would have a negative impact on standing balance; therefore a curvilinear relationship with P-CTSIB scores would be present. Linear regression incorporates only linear relationships into the model, therefore knee extension was eliminated.

Results

The isometric force output values for the right and left sides were combined for each muscle and are presented in Table 3. This was done to distinguish children with hemiplegia from children with diplegia. When the data are compared with results from typically developing children, the means are considerably lower (Hunt, 1994). Also presented in Table 3 is the percentage of limbs where children were unable to generate sufficient isometric force to register on the dynamometer. A dynamometer is a precise instrument that is reliable in children as young as three years of age (Gajdosik, 1994). The lack of force output, therefore, was attributed to subject weakness. Force output was 0 kilograms in 47% of limbs for hip flexion, 70% of limbs for knee flexion, and 21% of limbs for ankle dorsiflexion.

Descriptive statistics for range of motion are found in Table 4. Limitations were measured in every joint with the exception of foot inversion and eversion which frequently exceeded expected values. Joint movement with greatest range of motion limitation included hip flexion, hip abduction and ankle dorsiflexion.

Multiple regression analysis indicated that isometric muscle force and joint range of motion explained 54% of the variance in P-CTSIB scores (see Table 5). The children's lower extremity isometric muscle force explained 41% of the variance in P-CTSIB scores. Range of motion explained an additional 13% of the variance in P-CTSIB scores.

DISCUSSION

The results support the hypothesis that isometric muscle force and passive joint range of motion in the legs are predictors of standing balance abilities of children with CP who are able to walk. The variance in the subject's standing balance abilities explained by muscle force and range of motion is high (54%). This finding indicates that the greater the impairments in isometric muscle force and passive range, the greater the limitations in standing balance abilities of children with CP. In particular, isometric muscle force explained 41% of the variability in standing balance abilities. Weakness in ankle dorsiflexion and plantarflexion,

TABLE 3. Muscle Force Output Measured in Kilograms (N = 70 limbs) of Children with Cerebral Palsy

Movement	Minimum (%)*	Maximum	Mean	Median	Std. Deviation
Hip flexion	0 (47%)	10.2	1.3	.15	2.2
Hip extension	2.5	35.1	14.2	12.1	7.7
Hip abduction	0 (11%)	20.3	3.5	1.8	4.3
Knee flexion**	0 (70%)	8.2	.63	0	1.6
Knee extension**	0 (3%)	15.9	5.9	5.1	4.3
Dorsiflexion	0 (21%)	16.2	2.0	1.3	2.8
Plantarflexion	0 (3%)	27.6	10.1	9.4	7.3

* Percentage of limbs receiving this value
** N = 69

TABLE 4. Range of Motion Measured in Degrees (N = 70 limbs) of Children with Cerebral Palsy

Movement	Minimum	Maximum	Mean	Median	Std. Deviation
Hip flexion	84	140	116.8	120	15.2
Hip extension	−10	34	14.2	14	6.5
Hip abduction	0	58	32.4	31.5	11.7
Hip external rotation	14	86	52.4	55	12.7
Hip internal rotation	10	82	43.2	45.5	15.3
Knee flexion	62	158	140.0	144	15.4
Knee extension	166	194	180.8	180	6.0
Dorsiflexion	−14	40	13.5	12	9.2
Plantarflexion	18	50	35.2	35	7.4
Inversion	10	70	37.9	38	12.8
Eversion	14	60	36.9	37	10.3

TABLE 5. Results of Multiple Regression of Force and Range of Motion on P-CTSIB Scores

VARIABLE	R	R Square
Force Output	.64	.41
Range of Motion	.74	.54

df = 32

hip and knee extension, and hip abduction muscles may adversely influence standing balance. Strengthening the ankle muscles, increasing ankle range of motion or both may improve a child's ability to perform the "ankle strategy" typically seen in quiet stance or with small displacements in balance. Similarly, some children may need to increase hip extension force to perform a "hip strategy" used with larger displacements in standing.

The results must be interpreted carefully. Multiple regression analysis can detect relationships between variables, but a cause-effect relationship between isometric muscle force, passive joint range of motion and standing balance abilities in children with CP can not be inferred. Dynamic systems theory could not be directly tested in this study due to limitations in technology. The dynamic interplay between muscle force production and joint motion during the actual performance of standing balance activities was not measured. Instead, isometric muscle force and passive joint range of motion were measured to provide an indication of neuromuscular and musculoskeletal system impairments. Hand-held dynamometry measures isometric muscle contractions in prescribed testing positions while standing balance may use isometric, concentric and eccentric contractions at different joint angles. This puts the muscle at a different point on the length/tension curve and therefore changes the muscle's ability to generate force. The standing balance maneuvers require muscles to contract while in a weight bearing position while dynamometry utilizes non-weight bearing postures. Additionally, passive range of motion was measured rather than testing active range during the balance activity.

Implications for Clinical Practice

The results of this study, other research, and the authors' personal opinions provide the basis for several suggestions for clinical practice. Our suggestions apply only to children with CP who are similar to the subjects of this study (children 6 to 14 years of age with a Gross Motor Function Classification System level of I, II or III). We advocate that different interventions for improving standing balance abilities are needed for different children. The large ranges and standard deviations in the force data indicate that some of the children had much more weakness than others. The most effective methods of muscle strengthening for children with CP have not been determined. The magnitude of force production for standing balance abilities also has not been established.

Based on the results and our observations during testing, we recommend strengthening of ankle dorsiflexion and plantarflexion, and hip and knee extension muscles of children with CP. The large ranges and standard deviations in the force data indicate that some of the children had much more weakness than others. The results suggest that poor muscle force production may be a detrimental factor in standing balance of children with CP. This hypothesis is supported by research in typically developing children in which force production was shown to be the constraining factor for development of higher level upright movement skills, such as running, jumping, hopping, and skipping (Roncesvalles & Woollacott, 2000). Plantarflexor muscles spasticity should not be confused with strength, i.e., the ability to generate force in a useful manner (Damiano, Quinlivan, Owen, Shaffrey, & Abel, 2001; Fellows, Kaus, & Thilmann, 1994). At this time, the minimum value for the amount of ankle force needed for successful balance is not known. Since weakness is present in children with cerebral palsy, they may not be able to generate the force needed to perform an ankle strategy. Increasing ankle dorsiflexion and plantarflexion force production could aid the child in using an ankle strategy to make small postural adjustments to realign the center of mass within the base of support. A successful ankle strategy keeps the center of mass from moving further out towards the limits of stability and reduces the need for larger more dramatic balance maneuvers. Large balance maneuvers often require large compensations in the opposite direction and may be difficult for a child with CP to coordinate.

Crouched gait is another complex problem commonly seen in children with cerebral palsy. Hip and knee extension strengthening could potentially aid the child in assuming a more upright posture. The crouched standing posture affects the pattern of postural muscle coordination used to maintain balance. When children without motor disability are asked to adopt a crouched standing posture their postural motor coordination patterns became more similar to those of children with spastic diplegia (Woollacott, Burtner, & Jensen, 1998; Potter, Kirby, & MacLeod, 1990; Thorpe, Zaino, Westcott, & Valvano, 1998). By assuming a more erect posture, the child can use the normal biomechanical line of stability to help maintain stance. In the normal biomechanical line of stability, the line of gravity is slightly behind the hip joint and in front of the knee joint. The force of gravity creates an extension moment on these joints reducing the need for active muscle contraction during quiet stance. Additionally, adequate hip extension range of motion and force production would enable the child to use a hip strategy for maintaining balance.

Motor learning theory suggests that interventions should replicate the conditions of the functional task. Data on adults without neuromuscular abnormalities suggest that there is specificity of training in relation to the characteristics of the desired task such as the type, speed, and intensity of contraction and the weight bearing status during the contraction (Spielholz, 1990). We have interpreted this finding to suggest that balance should be practiced without orthotics in functional tasks that allow the muscle to work towards fatigue. To achieve a repetitive strong muscle contraction other limiting physical conditions may need to be modified. For example, if the child is unable to stand independently, a harness system would allow the child to walk for a longer time on the treadmill without stopping each time he lost his balance. Treadmill training with partial body weight support has been successful in improving performance on both the standing and walking sections of the Gross Motor Function Measure in a group of nonambulatory children with cerebral palsy (Schindl, Forstner, Kern, & Hesse, 2000). Walking in water with a flotation device might also provide prolonged exercise without falling.

Participation in community-based exercise and recreation programs could provide balance practice as well as improve overall levels of strength, fitness and motor planning. Programs such as gymnastics, tai chi, track, aerobics, and soccer provide opportunities to improve strength, endurance, peer interaction, and sportsmanship. Children of varying abilities can be accommodated through the use of adaptive equipment, physical assistance or environmental accommodation. Similar to children who are able bodied, emphasis should be placed on achieving a sustained level of physical activity to improve conditioning.

The authors' believe there is also a role for resistive exercise equipment, cuff weights, and theraband to increase force. It has been reported that children and adolescents with CP can increase force output through resistive exercise (Damiano, Quinlivan, Owen, Shaffrey, & Abel, 2001; Damiano, Kelly & Vaughn, 1995; Kramer & MacPhail, 1994; Parker, Carriere, Hebestreit, Salsberg, & Bar-Or, 1993; Shatsby & McCubbin, 1985). For children with severe weakness or severe motor incoordination, it may be difficult to sufficiently support the patient to allow repetitive strengthening through functional activities. Strengthening exercises may enable children to attain the minimum strength necessary for practice of functional activities. Specifically, the traditional training could improve the child's ability neurologically to activate the muscle, and then with functional movement against resistance, the muscle may then be able to show hypertrophy (Lieber, 1992; Lieber & Bodine-Fowler, 1993). At the other end of the spectrum, children with minimal or mild impairments in force production may not make improvements in strength through walking or other standing balance activities because the activities do not require the child to work towards muscle fatigue. Children with minimal or mild impairments may also benefit from traditional resistive exercise until they attain the strength needed to practice higher level motor skills. In both cases, however, we suggest that functional activities accompany traditional resistive exercise.

Similar to the arguments provided for functional strengthening, it is suggested that therapy interventions aimed at achieving active range of motion during a functional movement are more beneficial to the child than passive range of motion performed by a therapist. Adapted gymnastics, tai chi, karate, yoga, and dance are examples of activities a child could be asked to perform self stretching. Peer interaction could also promote tolerance of differences in children and adults through positive interaction with a child of differing abilities.

An important consideration for children with CP who are able to walk is the need for solid ankle foot orthotics. Limitations in ankle range of motion may preclude the use of balance strategies or may change the skeletal alignment and put the child at a gravitational disadvantage. For example, if dorsiflexion is significantly limited, the child may not be able to use an ankle strategy. Children in this study were observed barefoot and the most prevalent balance strategy attempted, although not always successful, was an ankle strategy. When children without motor impairments were constrained by wearing a solid ankle foot orthotics, postural motor patterns changed to resemble the patterns observed in children with CP wearing orthoses (Burtner, Woollacott, & Qualls, 1999). This finding suggests that solid ankle orthotics may preclude development of an effective ankle strategy. Additionally, immobilizing a muscle for prolonged periods of the day can lead to disuse atrophy and further weakness. We recommend children with CP who have some ankle mobility in standing perform physical activities on a regular basis without wearing orthotics.

Although wearing solid ankle orthotics may contribute to muscle weakness, the results for range of motion support stabilizing the foot. In general the children in this study had excessive foot eversion range of motion. The negative correlation between foot eversion range of motion and scores on the P-CTSIB ($-.367$, $p = .03$) indicates that as foot eversion range of motion increased, standing balance abilities decreased. This would suggest that limiting foot eversion range of motion may improve standing balance abilities. We advocate that orthotics to stabilize the midfoot be considered as part of a comprehensive intervention plan aimed at improving standing balance abilities. The recommended type of orthotics would incorporate a stable foot position such as those obtained through fabrication of a dynamic foot board and also would permit ankle movement. Ankle movement can be incorporated into an orthotic through the use of an ankle hinge or through a low profile orthotic that incorporates the foot and the malleoli, but that does not limit the ankle motion.

Conclusion/Clinical Impressions

The results provide evidence that isometric muscle force and passive joint range of motion are predictive of standing balance abilities in children with CP who are able to walk. The findings support examination of muscle strength and range of motion in the legs and evaluation of whether impairments are contributing to limitations in standing balance abilities. One single subject design pilot study examined the effects of strengthening on balance ability. The results were mixed, suggesting that individual clients may benefit more or less from the same intervention (Thawinchai, 2000). More research needs to be done to identify characteristics of children who benefit from support versus strength and movement at the ankles for improved balance and functional movement.

Future research that examines muscle force production and range of motion within the context of the functional activity would provide useful information about the minimum requirements necessary for maintaining adequate standing balance. Additionally, research is needed to determine the most effective interventions to improve muscle strength and range of motion in children with CP.

NOTE

1. Lafayette Instruments, 3700 Sagamore Parkway North, Lafayette, IN 47903.

REFERENCES

Atwater S. W., Crowe T. K., Deitz J. C., Richardson P.K. (1990). Interrater and test-retest reliability of two pediatric balance tests. *Physical Therapy, 70*, 79-87.

Bohannon R. W., Andrews A. W. (1987). Interrater reliability of hand-held dynamometry. *Physical Therapy, 6*, 931-933.

Bohannon R. W. (1986).Test-retest reliability of hand-held dynamometry during a single session of strength assessment. *Physical Therapy, 66*, 206-209.

Burtner P. A., Woollacott M. H., Shumway-Cook A. (1995). Muscle activation characteristics for balance control in children with cerebral palsy. *Developmental Medicine and Child Neurology, 37(S73)*, 27-28.

Burtner P. A., Qualls C. & Woollacott M. H. (1998). Muscle activation characteristics of stance balance control in children with spastic cerebral palsy. *Gait and Posture, 8*, 163-174.

Burtner P.A., Woollacott M.H., Qualls C. (1999). Stance balance control with orthoses in a group of children with spastic cerebral palsy. *Developmental Medicine and Child Neurology, 41*, 748-757.

Crowe T. K., Deitz J. C., Richardson P. K., Atwater S. W. (1990). Interrater reliability of the Clinical Test of Sensory Interaction for Balance. *Physical & Occupational Therapy in Pediatrics, 10*, 1-27.

Damiano D. L., Quinlivan J., Owen B. F., Shaffrey M., Abel M. F. (2001). Spasticity versus strength in cerebral palsy: Relationships among involuntary resistance, voluntary torque and motor function. *Eur J Neurol* Nov; 8 Suppl 5: 40-9.

Damiano D. L., Kelly L. E., Vaughn C. L. (1995). Effects of quadriceps femoris muscle strengthening on crouch gait in children with spastic diplegia. *Physical Therapy, 75,* 658-667.

Damiano D.L., Vaughan C.L., Abel M.F. (1995). Muscle response to heavy resistance exercise in children with spastic cerebral palsy. *Dev Med Child Neurol. 37,* 731-739.

Deitz J., Richardson P. K., Westcott S. L., Crowe T. K. (in press). Performance of children with learning disabilities on the Pediatric Clinical Test of Sensory Interaction for Balance. *Physical & Occupational Therapy in Pediatrics.*

Deitz J. C., Richardson P. K., Atwater S. W., Crowe T. K. (1991). Performance of normal children on the Pediatric Clinical Test of Sensory Interaction for Balance. *Occupational Therapy Journal of Research, 11,* 336-356.

Dichter C. G. (1994). Relationship of muscle strength and joint range of motion to gross motor abilities in school-aged children with Down syndrome. Unpublished doctoral dissertation. Medical College of Pennsylvania and Hahnemann University, Philadelphia, PA.

Dodd K.J., Taylor N.F., Damiano D.L. (2002). A systematic review of the effectiveness of strength-training programs for people with cerebral palsy. *Archives of Physical Medicine and Rehabilitation, 83 (8),* 1157-64.

Engsberg J.R., Ross S.A., Olree K.S., Park T.S. (2000). Ankle spasticity and strength in children with spastic diplegic cerebral palsy. *Developmental Medicine and Child Neurology, 42 (1)* 42-7.

Fellows S.J., Kau C., Thilmann A.F. (1994). Voluntary movement at the elbow in spastic hemiparesis. *Annals of Neurology, 36 (3).* 397-407.

Forssberg H., Nashner L. M. (1982). Ontogenetic development of postural control in man: Adaptation to altered support and visual conditions during stance. *Journal of Neuroscience, 2,* 545-552.

Foudriat B. A., DiFabio R. P., Anderson J. H. (1993). Sensory organization of balance responses in children 3-6 years age: A normative study with diagnostic implications. *International Journal of Pediatric Otorhinolarangology, 2,* 255-271.

Fowler E. G., Ho T. W., Nwige A. I., Dorey F. J. (2001). The effect of quadriceps femoris muscle strengthening exercises on spasticity in children with cerebral palsy. *Physical Therapy, 81 (6):* 1215-1223.

Gajdosik C. G., Nelson S. A., Gleason D. K. et al. (1994). Reliability of isometric strength measurements of girls ages 3-5 years: A preliminary study. *Pediatric Physical Therapy, 6,* 206.

Gajdosik R. L., Bohannon R. W. (1987). Clinical measurement of range of motion: Review of goniometry emphasizing reliability and validity. *Physical Therapy, 67,* 1867-1872.

Harris S. R., Harthun Smith L., Krukowski L. (1985). Goniometric reliability for a child with spastic quadriplegia. *Journal of Pediatric Orthopaedics, 5,* 348-351.

Horak F. B. (1987). Clinical measurement of postural control in adults. *Physical Therapy, 6,* 1881-1884.

Horvat M., Croce R., Roswal G. (1994). Intratester reliability of the Nicholas Manual Muscle Tester on individuals with intellectual disabilities by a tester having minimal experience. *Archives of Physical Medicine and Rehabilitation, 76*, 808-811.

Lowes L. P., Westcott S. L. (1995). Relationship of force output and range of motion to functional mobility tests in children with cerebral palsy. *Pediatric Physical Therapy, 7*, 200.

Palisano R. J., Rosenbaum P. L., Walter S. D., Russell D. J., Wood E. P., Galuppi B. E. (1997). Development and reliability of a system to classify gross motor function in children with cerebral palsy. *Developmental Medicine and Child Neurology, 39*, 214-223.

Parker D. F., Carriere L., Hebestreit H. et al. (1993). Muscle performance and gross motor function of children with spastic cerebral palsy. *Developmental Medicine and Child Neurology, 35*, 17-23.

Pelligrino T. T., Buelow B., Krause M., Loucks L. C., Westcott S. L. (1995). Test-retest reliability of the Pediatric Clinical Test of Sensory Interactions for Balance and the Functional Reach Test in children with standing balance dysfunction. *Pediatric Physical Therapy, 7*: 197.

Potter P.J., Kirby R.L., MacLeod D.A. (1990). The effects of simulated knee-flexion contractures on standing balance. *Amer J Phys Med Rehab. 69*, 144-147.

Richardson P. K., Atwater S. W., Crowe T. K., Deitz J. C. (1992). Performance of preschoolers on the Pediatric Clinical Test of Sensory Interaction for Balance. *American Journal of Occupational Therapy, 46*, 793-800.

Roncesvalles M.N., Woollacott M.H. (2000). The development of compensatory stepping skills in children. *Journal of Motor Behavior, 32*: 100-111.

Rose J., Haskell W.L., Gamble J.G., Hamilton R.L., Brown D.A., Rinsky L. (1994). *J Orthop Res.* Nov; 12 (6): 758-68.

Schindl M.R., Forstner C., Kern H., Hess S. (2000). Treadmill training with partial body weight support in nonambulatory patients with cerebral palsy. *Archives of Physical Medicine and Rehabilitation, 81 (3)*: 301-6.

Shumway-Cook A., Woollacott M. H. (1985). The growth of stability: Postural control from a developmental perspective. *Journal of Motor Behavior, 17*, 131-147.

Shumway-Cook A., & McCollum G. (1991). Assessment and treatment of balance deficits. In: Montgomery P. C., & Connolly B. H. (Eds.). Hixson, TN: Chattanooga Group Inc., 123-137.

Shumway-Cook A., Horak F. B. (1986). Assessing the influence of sensory interaction on balance: Suggestion from the field. *Physical Therapy, 66*, 1548-1550.

Shumway-Cook, A. & Woollacott M. H. (2001). *Motor Control: Theory and Practical Applications.* Baltimore: Lippincott, Wilkins & Williams.

Stuberg W. A., Fuchs R. H., Miedaner J. A. (1988). Reliability of goniometric measurements of children with cerebral palsy. *Developmental Medicine and Child Neurology, 30*, 657-666.

Thorpe D., Westcott S. L. (1998). Comparison of postural muscle coordination patterns during a functional reaching task in typically developing children and children with cerebral palsy. *Physical Therapy, 78:* S80-81.

Thorpe D., Zaino C., Westcott S., & Valvano J. (1998). Comparison of postural muscle coordination patterns during a functional reaching task in typically developing children and children with cerebral palsy. *Physical Therapy, 78,* S80-81.

Westcott S. L., Crowe T. K., Deitz J. C., Richardson P. K. (1994). Test-retest reliability of the Pediatric Clinical Test of Sensory Interaction for Balance (P-CTSIB). *Physical & Occupational Therapy in Pediatrics, 14:* 1-22.

Westcott S. L., Lowes L. P., Richardson P. K. (1997). Evaluation of postural stability in children: Current theories and assessment tools. *Physical Therapy, 77:* 629-645.

Woollacott M. H., Shumway-Cook A. (1990). Changes in posture control across the life span–A systems approach. *Physical Therapy, 70,* 799-807.

Woollacott M. H., Burtner P., Jensen J. L. (1998). Development of postural responses during standing in healthy children and children with spastic diplegia. *Neurosci Biobehav, 22:* 583-589.

World Health Organization. (2001). *International Classification of Functioning, Disability, and Health (ICF)* Geneva: World Health Organization.

Activity-Focused Motor Interventions
for Children with Neurological Conditions

Joanne Valvano

SUMMARY. This article presents a model to guide activity-focused physical therapy and occupational therapy interventions for children with neurological conditions. Activity-focused interventions involve structured practice and repetition of functional actions and are directed toward the learning of motor tasks that will increase independence and participation in daily routines.

According to this model, the pediatric therapist: (1) develops activity-related goals in collaboration with the child and the family; (2) plans activity-focused interventions by adapting knowledge of motor learning to the child's individual learning strengths and needs; and (3) integrates impairment-focused intervention with activity-focused intervention. *[Article copies available for a fee from The Haworth Document Delivery Service: 1-800-HAWORTH. E-mail address: <docdelivery@haworthpress.com> Website: <http://www.HaworthPress.com> © 2004 by The Haworth Press, Inc. All rights reserved.]*

KEYWORDS. Neurological disorders, cerebral palsy, physical therapy intervention, occupational therapy intervention, motor learning

---

Joanne Valvano, PT, PhD, is affiliated with Physical Therapy Program, University of Colorado Health Sciences Center, 4200 East Ninth Avenue, C244, Denver, CO 80262 (E-mail: Joanne.Valvano@UCHSC.edu).

[Haworth co-indexing entry note]: "Activity-Focused Motor Interventions for Children with Neurological Conditions." Valvano, Joanne. Co-published simultaneously in *Physical & Occupational Therapy in Pediatrics* (The Haworth Press, Inc.) Vol. 24, No. 1/2, 2004, pp. 79-107; and: *Movement Sciences: Transfer of Knowledge into Pediatric Therapy Practice* (ed: Robert J. Palisano) The Haworth Press, Inc., 2004, pp. 79-107. Single or multiple copies of this article are available for a fee from The Haworth Document Delivery Service [1-800-HAWORTH, 9:00 a.m. - 5:00 p.m. (EST). E-mail address: docdelivery@haworthpress.com].

Current physical therapy and occupational therapy interventions for children with neurological conditions emphasize the learning or re-learning of motor tasks that increase independence and participation in daily routines (Ketelaar, Vermeer, Hart, Van Petegem-van Beek & Helders, 2001; Larin, 2000; McEwen & Sheldon, 1995). Activity-fo-cused interventions involve structured practice and repetition of func-tional tasks to promote learning. Motor learning theory provides the foundation for these interventions. It supports guidelines for structuring practice in ways that enhance the learning and generalization of motor activities. Motor learning content is increasingly being integrated into the curricula for occupational therapy and physical therapy education programs and the theoretical basis for intervention (Heriza & Sweeney, 1994). However, there is a discontinuity, in that pediatric therapists re-port difficulty with effectively integrating motor learning principles into their intervention strategies. In a survey of pediatric physical thera-pists, about 70% of the respondents reported that they would like to im-plement motor learning concepts in their interventions for children with disability, but they required more information to practically apply them (Hayes, McEwen, Lovett, Sheldon, & Smith, 1999).

I propose that motor learning principles would be a more natural fit for therapy interventions, if they were complemented by a methodology to address impairments in body functions and structures that affect mo-tor learning. Neurological impairments that affect motor learning can be addressed in two ways: (1) adapting motor learning guidelines to meet the individual learning challenges of the young learner; and (2) integrat-ing activity-focused interventions with interventions focused on im-pairments. According to the International Classification of Functioning, Disability, and Health (World Health Organization, 2001), impairments are problems in physiologic functions of the body or anatomic struc-tures. Impairments can be temporary or permanent, static or progres-sive, and may lead to other impairments. Impairments place limits on functional activity and participation in life's roles.

More empirical data are needed to assist the practitioner in applying motor learning guidelines to the practice of motor skills (Duff & Quinn, 2000; Larin, 2000). In some cases, these guidelines may require adapta-tion to meet the individual learning needs of children with neurological impairments. The motor learning paradigms that are used to generate guidelines for conducting practice often involve simple experimental tasks, not complex functional tasks that children need to function in the natural environment. The natural environment is also more complex than the experimental environment. Experimental tasks, such as tapping tasks or linear positioning tasks, may require the capable subject to meet timing or accuracy requirements of a movement that is already in the repertoire of the subject (Schmidt & Wrisberg, 2000). Children with neurological conditions often must acquire the basic coordination of the movement required to achieve a functional motor task. Furthermore, sensory and motor functions, which are taken for granted in most motor learning paradigms, can be impaired in children with neurological conditions.

Systematically integrating impairment-focused interventions with activity-focused interventions should also enhance the application of motor learning approaches. There may be a misconception among therapists, that impairment-focused interventions are not compatible with intervention approaches that emphasize motor learning. Physical therapists and occupational therapists consider impairment-focused interventions to be important. Primary impairments, such as spasticity, might be targets for medical or surgical interventions, such as botulinum toxin A injection or dorsal rhizotomy. Secondary impairments that develop over time, such as joint contractures, muscle weakness, or poor endurance, are often the focus of physical therapy and occupational therapy interventions because they affect the performance and learning of functional activities. Furthermore, secondary impairments are the targets of preventive interventions, which limit the degree of disability associated with these impairments in body structures and functions. (Bartlett & Palisano, 2002; *Guide to Physical Therapist Practice,* 2001).

The purpose of this paper is to present a model of intervention for children with neurological conditions that gives primacy to practice that supports the learning of functional motor activity, but also addresses impairments associated with neurological diagnoses. This framework should assist clinical reasoning regarding motor learning interventions, and provide a structure for scientific inquiry.

MODEL OF INTERVENTION

Figure 1 depicts a model for motor learning interventions, which emphasizes the learning and generalization of functional motor tasks. Interventions are categorized into *activity-focused* and *impairment-focused.* Activity-focused interventions involve structured practice and repetition of functional actions. Guidelines for conducting practice from the motor learning literature provide the foundation for organizing the task and the environment to maximize learning. These guidelines are adapted, when necessary, to meet the individual learning strengths and needs of the young learner. Impairment-focused interventions are directed toward ameliorating the effects of impairments in body structures and functions associated with neurological conditions and preventing secondary impairments from developing.

Theoretical Framework for Model

Dynamic Systems Perspective

The intervention model presented in this paper borrows metaphors about change from the dynamic systems perspective on motor learning. Dynamic concepts about change are derived from Bernstein's study of the organization of movement (Bernstein, 1967) and mathematical methods of the dynamic pattern theory (Haken, Kelso & Bunz, 1985; Scholz, 1990).

FIGURE 1. Model of Interventions for Children with Neurological Disorders, Which Integrates Activity-Focused Interventions with Impairment-Focused Interventions by Physical Therapist or Occupational Therapist as Change Agent

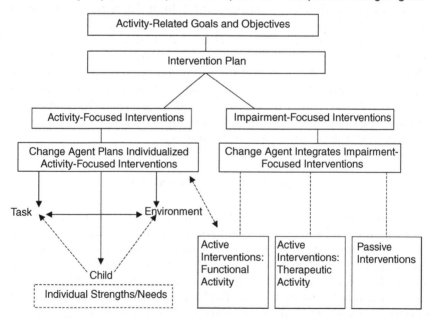

Basically, motor learning involves a change or transition to a new motor behavior. In order for functional change to occur, a new, preferred coordination must replace the former (Kelso, 1984; Scholz & Kelso, 1990; Newell, 1996; Newell & Valvano, 1998; Zanone & Kelso, 1991). The term *coordination* refers to the organization of degrees of freedom into a behavioral unit, which therapists might call a pattern of movement. Qualitative aspects of coordination describe the form of the movement, or the relationship of the body segments to one another. Quantitative aspects of coordination describe the refinement or scaling of the basic pattern to meet task requirements. Examples of quantitative aspects of coordination are speed, magnitude or timing of the movement (Newell, 1996). The preferred coordination that a child demonstrates is determined by the intrinsic coordination tendencies. These tendencies, or dynamics, are a function of a complex movement system, composed of multiple, interacting subsystems, within a specified task and environmental context (Newell, 1996; Zanone, Kelso, & Jeka, 1993).

In the course of infant development, changes in functional motor behaviors, such as reaching, and locomotion, occur as infants engage in exploration. Progression in each of the component systems alters the intrinsic coordination tendencies of the infant and new, preferred patterns of movement emerge (Heriza, 1991; Zanone, Kelso, & Jeka, 1993). Thelan (1986) outlined the changes in contributing systems (including motivation, strength, tonus control and body characteristics) that induce the transition to independent stepping as the preferred locomotor behavior in infants. These component systems, along with the task requirements and the environmental context, act as control parameters to induce developmental change. In dynamic pattern theory, a control parameter is a critical variable, which provides conditions for change, as it takes on a critical state or value.

Infants with neurological disorders may not show the desired progression of one or more subsystems. To support desired developmental change in these infants, the change agent focuses on the systems that limit developmental change and organizes features of the task and environment that induce the desired motor behavior (Heriza, 1991). The intervention model depicted in Figure 1 can be applied to interventions with infants. However, the content of this paper, in the sections that follow, will focus on intentional, verbally mediated practice by children.

During goal-directed practice, manipulation of a control parameter can induce a spontaneous change in motor behavior, if the required coordination mode is available. Recall that control parameters may reside in the task, the environment, or in the multiple components of the child's complex movement system. Spontaneous change in motor behavior has been studied through experimental bimanual finger tapping tasks (Kelso, 1984). A change in coordination from the anti-phase (the range of index finger abduction and adduction on one hand is 180° out of phase with the other) to in-phase tapping spontaneously occurs when the frequency requirements of the experimental task increase to a critical point. The in-phase tapping is more stable and preferred at high frequencies, given the coordination tendencies of adult performers.

The coordination required to perform a new functional activity is often not available to the learner. Impairments in component systems can limit the coordination repertoire of children with neurological conditions. Functional change, in these cases, requires effort, and intentional, goal-directed practice with feedback and other behavioral information (Scholz, 1990). A new coordination pattern must be learned. Studies of intentional learning processes, using simple experimental movements, have led to some dynamic principles about learning that can be applied to activity-focused interventions (Scholz & Kelso, 1989, 1990; Smethurst & Carson, 2003). First, the effect of practice relates to the stability (the resistance to change) of the current movement patterns. Practice may have a diminished effect if the existing pattern of movement is very stable, or resistant to change. This principle suggests that practice interventions may be more successful during periods of change or fluctuations in component systems (e.g., the period of biomechanical change after orthopedic surgery or botulinum toxin injections) because these fluctuations make the behavior more likely to change. Second, the effect of practice, or the likelihood of change, is affected by the degree to which the requirements of the to-be-learned behavior are different from the current behavior (Scholz, 1990; Scholz & Kelso, 1990; Wenderoth, Bock & Krohn, 2002; Zanone & Kelso, 1991). These concepts can be applied to the process or prognosis, which requires the therapist to anticipate the potential for progress in developing goals for the Plan of Care (*Guide to Physical Therapist Practice*, 2001).

Learning a novel task, such as juggling for a child with typical development or ascending stairs for a child with cerebral palsy, involves an active search for a solution to a movement problem (Scholz, 1990; Newell, 1996; Newell & Valvano, 1998). This concept is essential to the model presented here because it defines the role of the physical therapist or occupational therapist as a change agent who facilitates the child's search for a coordination solution that will enable a task to be performed or refined. The concept of constraints on action is also essential to this model.

Constraints are factors related to the performer, the task, and the environment (or context of learning) that interact with each other to influence the outcome of a movement experience. This concept of constraints applies the concept of the control parameter from dynamic pattern theory to practical or clinical learning situations (Clark, 1995; Majak, 1996; Newell & Valvano, 1998). These factors are called constraints because they limit or constrain the possible movement outcomes that might emerge as the child attempts to achieve an action. Constraints can be enablers or positive influence to learning (because they restrict the possible outcomes to positive ones) or limiters to learning (because they inhibit change or support the outcome that is not desired). In this model, the change agent interacts with the triad of constraints (task, the environment and the child) to facilitate the desired outcome of practice (Newell & Valvano, 1998). This interaction of constraints is depicted by the triangle in Figure 1. This process of modifying constraints of the task and environment is aided by practice guidelines from the motor learning literature. The change agent addresses personal constraints by identifying strengths as well as impairments that affect learning.

Practice, from a dynamic systems perspective, was illustrated in our work with children with spastic diplegia, who learned to move a therapeutic exercise scooter backward (Valvano, Heriza & Carollo, 2003). The task requires the children to stand, hands supported on vertical uprights, with each foot on a platform. The child displaces the platforms, which move the wheels, by shifting weight and alternating leg flexion and extension. Kinematic analysis revealed that, after repeated practice trials, the coordination of certain segments, including the ankle and pelvis changed. As task-related patterns of movement emerged, the task of moving the scooter was accomplished. After continued practice, the basic coordination improved and the functional outcome was characterized by increased speed and efficiency. We modified task constraints, such as the duration of the trial and the position of the feet on the platforms as well as environment constraints, such as the floor surface, and the hand supports, to increase the child's success. We experimented with verbal and physical guidance as a way to modify the informational constraints and support successful learning.

Information Processing Perspective

Many of the task and environment-related guidelines from the motor learning literature are based on principles from the information processing perspective. The assumptions of the information processing perspective, which emphasize cognitive aspects of motor learning and abstract memory representations (motor programs), are quite different from those of the dynamic systems perspective. However, cognitive and memory systems are certainly among the many contributing systems that determine the outcome of motor activity. Principle concepts from the information processing perspective are: (a) the proposed stages of information processing that occur prior to movement execution, (b) memory, and (c) attention. These information processing stages affect reaction time, which is the duration in time between the presentation of an environmental stimulus or the intent to move, and the actual initiation of the movement response. The slow, awkward quality of movement seen in children with neurological conditions may be accounted for by information processing deficits in addition to limitations in the production of movement.

Memory functions obviously are important to enable the learner to benefit from prior experience. Motor learning guidelines, related to the task and environment, enhance long-term retention and generalization of motor skills by emphasizing active processes that encode information into long-term memory for future retrieval. Some children with cerebral palsy have been identified to have deficits in motor memory, which affects the development of motor plans that can be retrieved for functional motor activity (Lesny et al., 1990).

The final construct from the information processing approach is attention, which can be defined as the focusing of information processing resources. Selective attention is critical for extracting the relevant information in the environment for task performance (Light, 1991; Schmidt & Wrisberg, 2000). Another application of attention to motor learning is the assumption that there is a limited capacity of attention. That is, children can basically concentrate on a limited amount of information at one time. Even well-learned tasks, such as walking, can be affected by the interference of a secondary cognitive task in young children (Huang, Mercer & Thorpe, 2003). We know that, in natural environments, like the classroom, children are required to focus on many things at once. Basically, the interference that a competing task has with the primary task depends on how well learned or automatic the primary task is. If the primary task is well learned and automatic, it doesn't require as many attention resources (Huang & Mercer, 2001; Schmidt & Wrisberg, 2000). Therefore, resources are available for secondary or tertiary tasks.

Practical Steps for Intervention

The practical steps in this model for intervention are:

1. Develop *activity-related goals* and *objectives* that will increase participation and quality of life, based on priorities of the child and family, in collaboration with the intervention team.
2. Plan *activity-focused intervention* by: (1) identifying environment and task modifications based on motor learning principles (2) adapting these practice guidelines, when necessary, to address constraints of the child, in terms of individual learning strengths and needs.
3. Integrate *impairment-focused intervention* with activity-focused intervention. These can be executed in the context of goal-related functional activity or executed outside of the context of functional activity.

These practical steps in the intervention process will be discussed in the sections that follow, with application primarily to cerebral palsy and reference to a case study of a child with spastic diplegia.

Case Study

Clara is a first grade student, 7 years, 1 month of age. She has the diagnosis of spastic diplegia. She was born prematurely at 32 weeks and experienced complications of prematurity, including a Grade 3 intraventricular hemorrhage. Clara's functional level would be classified as Level 3, according to the Gross Motor Function Classification System (Palisano, Rosenbaum, Walter, Russell, Wood, & Galuppi, 1997). Clara has independent functional mobility in the home without use of assistive aids, but she does not walk steadily enough to be an independent community ambulator. For safety in the classroom and in the community, Clara uses a four-wheeled reverse rollator walker and bilateral hinged ankle-foot orthoses. She receives physical therapy services in the school, which are complemented by weekly sessions in an outpatient physical therapy clinic. Clara's physical therapist and parents have begun practice of walking, using a single forearm crutch. She ascends and descends stairs, with supervision, using two handrails. She has a "stiff-knee gait" (Gage, 1991), with reduced knee flexion in swing. In barefoot walking, there is a toe-toe gait pattern on initial contact. There is marked internal rotation of the leg during locomotor activity.

Strength in the lower extremities is in the poor to fair range, except for near-normal strength in the quadriceps. There is significant pelvic instability in upright skills and single leg stance is challenging. There are no significant limitations in joint range of motion. She had percutaneous hamstring releases two years ago and range of motion has been maintained. There is significant increase in dynamic tone, with bias toward extension, when Clara engages in upright activity.

Activity-Related Goals

Developing activity-related goals is the first step in developing intervention plans that will increase independence and participation for children with neurological movement conditions. According to current "top-down" approaches (Campbell, 1991), goals related to functional outcomes are determined first. Then, components that limit these outcomes are assessed. The emphasis on activity-focused intervention is in contrast to more traditional interventions that have, in the past, focused on the impairments that limit functional activity (Heriza & Sweeney, 1994). Activity-focused interventions are in compliance with the Individual with Disabilities Education Act, which mandates the development of educational plans that encourage individuals with neurological disability to become productive members of the community and to function in the school environment. Recent advances in neurosciences, which suggest that coordination and motor control emerge in the context of functional tasks, also support activity-oriented approaches (Horak, 1991; Hadders-Algra, 2000).

To increase participation at school and at her grandmother's home (where stair-cases have only one railing), Clara's parents would like her to learn to ascend and descend stairs, independently, using one railing. The stated goal is: Clara will ascend or descend a flight of 10 stairs, with supervision only, using one handrail in two minutes or less, 100% of the time. The practice goal, set up for the immediate practice sessions, is to ascend three stairs independently, using one handrail, in 30 seconds.

Activity-Focused Intervention

According to the International Classification of Function, Disability and Health (WHO, 2001), activity is the performance of a task or action. Action implies intention and a strategy to achieve a functional goal (Gentile, 1992; Newell & Valvano, 1998). In activity-focused interventions, the change agent plans activity to support the target functional motor behavior. Practice of functional activity is the most important motor learning variable (Schmidt & Wrisberg, 2000) and evidence is emerging for the benefits of intentional practice by children with neurological conditions (Gordon & Duff, 1999; Thorpe & Valvano, 2001; Valvano, Heriza & Carollo, 2003; Valvano & Newell, 1998).

To achieve the goal specified in a child's intervention plan, the change agent may structure practice of the target activity, in this case, ascending stairs with one railing. The practice of the target task is often complemented by practice of tasks that share common elements or components. For example, Clara might practice stepping and climbing on playground equipment. Therapists often use a variety of related tasks because of the practical limitations of having young children perform increased trials of the same target task.

The extent to which components of movement practiced in a related activity transfer to the target functional activity requires empirical study. In general, motor learning theory predicts a small amount of transfer between tasks, so practice of the target skill is recommended (Schmidt & Wrisberg, 2000; Winstein, Gardner, McNeal, Barto & Nicholson, 1989). However, practice of related tasks, which focus on shared movement components, may play an increased role in motor learning by children with neurological disorders, who have a limited coordination repertoire. Horne, Warren and Jones (1995) reported that children, from 21 to 34 months of age, who practiced activities that targeted specific movement components, were able to increase the performance of the targeted activity and generalize the movement components to untreated exemplar activities. For children with cognitive limitations, practice of prerequisite skills may not be advisable because of difficulty with transfer to the target task (McEwen, 2000).

I would like to make two points, related to practice of functional activities, which address components of movement.

1. *The focus of practice should be on the action, not the patterns of movement.* The child's efforts to meet task requirements drive the change in motor patterns. Van der Weel and colleagues (Van der Weel, van der Meer, & Lee, 1991) evaluated the component of forearm supination in children with CP. This movement is difficult for children who demonstrate a flexion pattern in the upper extremity. The experiment demonstrated that increased active supination was achieved when the children used the limb to perform a functional action, beating on a drum, compared to when

they practiced the movement of supination. The task gave meaning and a goal structure to the movement pattern.

2. *Normal movement quality is not the goal of practice.* The change agent structures opportunities for learning a functional task. A task can be achieved through many different means and preferred coordination patterns are individual, based on the child's unique movement capabilities (Bernstein, 1967; Newell, 1996; Valvano & Newell, 1998). However, if the child chooses a coordination mode that brings about an unsuccessful or unsafe outcome, the change agent directs the child to a more appropriate pattern, based on analysis of the task (Newell & Valvano, 1998). Likewise, if the preferred pattern can cause secondary complications over time, the therapist may direct the child to a different pattern (Darrah & Bartlett, 1995). On the other hand, therapists must be careful about making decisions about efficiency based on qualitative aspects of the child's movement (Darrah & Bartlett, 1995). I know a golfer who has a terrible swing, but hits the ball 250 yards. We found that some children with cerebral palsy demonstrate better performance on an isometric grip force task using preferred forearm and wrist patterns that were "atypical," compared to when the forearm and wrist were supported in typical postures (Valvano & Newell, 1998).

Clara currently cannot achieve the functional task of ascending stairs, using one railing, using her preferred coordination pattern. She primarily relies on pulling herself up to the next step, using the upper extremities. The reliance on the arm strategy increases trunk and pelvis hyperextension, which increases the difficulty with controlled and timely flexion of the leg to clear the step and place the advancing foot. In this case, she is guided to explore a strategy which modifies hand placement on the railings encourages the weight to advance forward.

According to the model in Figure 1, the therapeutic activity-focused interventions are planned according to motor learning guidelines with consideration of the strengths and learning needs of the individual child. This process involves the following practical steps:

1. *Identify the child's strengths and limitations* that might affect the process of motor learning. These limitations are associated with impairments in functions and structures of the multiple interacting systems. Certain systems may be of greater importance for some children. In the section that follows, limitations in the sensory and motor systems will be discussed.

2. *Identify special learning needs* through analysis of how impairments impact on varied mechanisms that are important for the process of motor learning. These mechanisms include information processing, error detection, feed-forward performance, and automatic performance.
3. *Apply guidelines for practice* from the motor learning literature, related to the *task* and the *environment*. Apply these guidelines directly where appropriate. Make adaptations, when indicated, to account for special learning needs.

Identification of Impairments That Influence the Process of Motor Learning

Although the strengths of the learner are critical to the process of learning, this section will address impairments in sensory and motor functions that might limit the motor learning process. Recall that sensory and motor systems are among the multiple components of the child's complex movement system. However, before proceeding to the discussion of special learning needs, I should discuss developmental factors, which are critical for goal setting and planning therapeutic practice. The knowledge of sensory-motor development as well as development of cognitive functions is important in planning activity-focused interventions. Planning for the psychosocial environment, as it relates to the therapist-child relationship, depends on the developmental level of the learner. Larin (2000) discusses the concept of therapeutic power in the session and the decisions the therapist makes about sharing the decision-making. The roles of the therapist as instructor and playmate are balanced to meet the child's needs and the productivity of the session. In the case of Clara, the therapist allows Clara to engage in imaginative play, which gives meaning to the stairs task and makes the practice fun for her.

Impairments in Sensory Processing

Impairments in visual-perception (Lee & Cook, 1990; Stiers, Vanderkelen, Vanneste, Coene, De Rammelacre & Vandenbussche, 2002) affect the process of motor learning. For Clara, impaired visual processing could contribute to her difficulty with accurate placing the foot on the step. Howard and Henderson (1989) examined deficits in visual perception relative to functional mobility. Children with spastic and athetoid cerebral palsy were asked to make height and weight judgments about their ability to pass through a door-shaped aperture, which was systematically changed. The children with spastic cerebral palsy were significantly less accurate than children with athetosis and children with no neurodevelopmental impairments in their judgments.

Impairments in visual processing may be affected by the reduced range and amount of motor activity experienced by children with neurological conditions. They have limited practice with appreciating salient visual information from the environment and matching perceptual requirements with an efficient movement response (Goodgold-Edwards & Gianutsis, 1991; Sugden & Keogh, 1990).

Somatosensory processing may also be impaired in children with cerebral palsy (Blanche & Nakasuji, 2000; Eliasson, Gordon, & Forssberg, 1992, 1995). Clara's reliance on vision for foot placement on the step and apparent lack of ability to detect errors in foot placement suggest that impaired proprioceptive awareness may contribute to limitations in locomotion as well as the stair task.

Impairments in Motor Production

Sugden and Keogh (1990) summarize motor production deficits in children with CP in terms of impairments in motor unit control and use of poorly differentiated synergistic movement patterns. Impaired force production is central to the motor control disorder of children with cerebral palsy. Force production relies on neural control of muscle activation patterns, which determine the selection, timing, sequencing, and magnitude of muscle activity. Impairments in selective muscle activity are compounded by impairments in strength and endurance, as well as musculoskeletal impairments.

When Clara ascends stairs, there is reduced postural control, force production and selective control of leg flexion. Movement of the tibia over the foot of the advancing leg is difficult, due to hypoextensibility.

Identify Special Learning Needs

Impairments in sensory integration and motor production associated with neurological conditions give rise to special learning needs that can affect the process of motor learning and the application of practice guidelines from the motor learning literature. Special learning needs will be described below, in terms of selected mechanisms of motor learning.

Information Processing

Information processing has been a focus of research on motor learning. The stages of information processing described by Schmidt (1988) are: (a) *stimulus identification* which involves selectively attending to and interpreting relevant stimuli about the task from the environment; (b) *response selection*, which involves choosing a suitable motor response; and (c) *response programming* which, theoretically, organizes the response in the central nervous system before movement is initiated. The dynamic systems perspective emphasizes the natural linkage of the child's movements with the environment.

Reaction time is a measure of the speed of information processing time. Parks, Rose and Dunn (1989) reported that children with left spastic hemiplegia required significantly more time to plan (not execute) a simple aiming movement with the right hand, compared to children with no disability. Information processing limitations can account for slow, inefficient movement.

Disorders in sensory processes complicate mechanisms of information processing. Research on precision grip by children with hemiplegic cerebral palsy illustrates limitations in matching sensory properties of objects with efficient motor responses (Eliasson, Gordon & Forssberg, 1991). Children with typical development use grip forces that are precisely scaled to match the weight and surface properties of an object. On the other hand, children with CP used overall-high grip forces and did not adjust to properties of the object in a systematic way. Impairments in motor production increase the complexity of tasks for children with cerebral palsy. Complexity of the motor response is one factor that increases information processing requirements and the reaction time (Christina, 1982).

Error Detection

Clara's therapist suspects that error detection may limit Clara's learning to control her posture and foot placement, even after repeated trials. Error detection is critical to motor learning. Harbourne (2001) compared the ability of adolescents with cerebral palsy with the ability of adolescents with typical development to accurately achieve a target speed of upper extremity movement and the detect errors. The speed error relative to the target was significantly increased and the ability to detect errors was significantly reduced for the children with cerebral palsy. There was great variability in the error detection capability, which was not related to degree of motor involvement. Error detection depends on intrinsic feedback as well as extrinsic feedback provided by the change agent.

Motor performance of children with cerebral palsy is characterized by high inter-trial variability (Eliasson, Gordon & Forssberg, 1991, 1992; Thorpe & Valvano, 2002; Valvano & Newell, 1995; Valvano, Westcott & Palisano, 1998). Children with cerebral palsy often do not demonstrate the orderly improvement in performance over practice trials commonly seen in children with typical development. This inconsistency among trials of practice could affect the mechanisms of error detection during the iterative process of practice.

Feedforward Performance

Clara relies on visual input to judge the degree of leg flexion required to clear the step with the advancing leg and to place the foot on the step. This slows her movement down considerably. Contrast this behavior with the child who speedily runs up the steps without on-line feedback about the range of leg movement required to clear the step. This scenario describes feedforward mechanisms, which do not rely on ongoing sensory input. Movements are performed with anticipation of the sensory requirements for the action and are faster because they do not depend on the processing of external sensory information. Feedback and feedforward mechanisms complement each other in skilled movement. Children with cerebral palsy may not develop a plan of action and feedforward control as capably as their typically developing peers (Bly, 1996; Eliasson, Gordon, & Forssberg, 1992; Parks, Rose, & Dunn, 1989; Valvano, Heriza, & Carollo, 2002).

The challenges in developing feedforward control in children with cerebral palsy are depicted by a series of studies of grip force. After lifting an object a few times, the children with typical development planned in advance, or anticipated, the grip force requirement prior to lift the object. On the other hand, the children with cerebral palsy were more reliant on somatosensory feedback from the object to grade grip forces. They required predictable conditions and many more trials to develop the memory representation required to anticipate the grip force requirements. The reliance on feedback contributes to the awkward quality of manipulative functions (Eliasson, Gordon, & Forssberg, 1992; Gordon & Duff, 1999).

Yao (1995) studied the perception-action match in children with cerebral palsy through the investigation of pre-shaping of the aperture between the thumb and index finger, prior to gripping three sizes of objects. Children with typical development systematically scaled the aperture to the size of the object, prior to lift. Children with cerebral palsy did not systematically adjust aperture prior to lift. The anticipation of the aperture can be considered a feedforward mechanism.

Somatosensory impairments may contribute to the delayed development of feedforward control (Eliasson et al., 1991, 1992). Development of feedforward mechanisms depends on reliable sensory consequences of actions, such as of the height of stepping. They also rely on predictable, controlled motor responses (Blanche & Nakusuji, 2000).

Automatic Performance

Even when Clara ascends the stairs with two railings, her performance becomes less reliable and safe when she attends to conversations or other events in the environment. The interference from a concurrent task is increased when the primary task is not automatic. Automatic performance is quick, error free, consistent, and allows attention resources to be allocated to competing tasks in the natural environment. Developmental considerations and the information processing limitations of children with neurological conditions may place limits on automatic performance in the natural environment (Huang & Mercer, 2001; Huang, Mercer, & Thorpe, 2003).

Adapt Motor Learning Guidelines to Enhance Practice

Practice guidelines are intended to enhance to benefits of practice, thereby promoting the retention and generalization of the motor behavior. From a dynamic system perspective, the new behavior becomes more stable. Task-related interventions relate to the content, structure, or schedule of presentation of the task. Environment-related interventions include the physical environment, the psychosocial environment, and the performance environment (Heriza, 1991). The performance environment is characterized by the augmented information provided to the learner by the change agent. Augmented information, such as feedback and guidance, complements intrinsic information naturally available to the child upon performance of the task.

Decisions about motor learning guidelines take the stage of learning into account. In the early stages, the learner discovers the conditions that must be met in order to successfully achieve the task and a possible coordination strategy to achieve the goal. In the later stages of practice, the learner develops skill, the coordination is refined and the movement becomes efficient (Gentile, 1999).

Practice guidelines based on motor learning research may be directly applicable to practice by children with neurological conditions and require no adaptation. In some cases, however, guidelines may require adaptation to meet special learning needs related to mechanisms of motor learning. To address special learning needs, the change agent may: (a) *enhance* motor learning guidelines, or (b) *modify* motor learning guidelines. Strategies to *enhance* practice guidelines involve applying the guidelines, but augmenting their application by strategies to increase effectiveness. Strategies to *modify* practice guidelines, involve altering their application based on the child's special learning needs.

Research regarding to identify optimal practice strategies and adaptations is essential for activity-focused intervention. Even in the absence of a systematic body of evidence, therapists should contemplate a child's learning strengths and learning challenges and individualize guidelines for practice accordingly. Adapting practice guidelines to address special learning needs of children with neurological conditions will be illustrated according to two categories of practice variables from the motor learning literature: task-related guidelines and guidelines related to augmented information.

Task-Related Guidelines

Variable versus constant structure of practice is an example of a practice guideline that might be adapted to meet individual needs. With variable or varied practice, the task is structured to allow the child to rehearse a number of variations of a task during the session. Constant practice involves rehearsal of only one variation of a task in a session. Variable practice has been shown to be more effective than constant practice in performing novel movement variations by children (Carson & Wigand, 1979; Wulf, 1991). The ability to generalize the movement to many situations, including novel situations, is important for children with cerebral palsy who must apply movement skills to the school and community environments. Table 1 lists examples of adaptations to variable practice and related special learning needs, based on components of motor learning. These have not been empirically tested.

Guidelines Related to Augmented Information: Instruction and Feedback

Providing augmented information is a primary task of the change agent during practice. I will address instruction provided prior to prac-

TABLE 1. Proposed Adaptations to Variable Practice and Related Special Learning Needs

Proposed Adaptation to Variable Practice	Special Learning Need Related to Motor Learning Mechanism
Enhance the benefits of variable practice by helping the child cue into the relevant features of the task variation (e.g., the height of the steps, the position of the railing). Cueing helps the child to anticipate the proper movement response. **Enhance** effects of variable practice by providing many trials and many exemplars to enhance generalization.	Ability to identify the task relevant information that is required for generalizing may not be well developed, due to **information processing limitations**.
Modify the variable practice schedule to a "constant-variable" practice schedule. Provide constant practice initially, then progress to variable practice.	Early in practice, **information processing** resources are devoted to developing the basic coordination requirement. Therefore, the advantages of variable practice may not be beneficial until the later phases of practice, after the basic coordination of the movement has been achieved. Early phases of practice are prolonged, due to learning needs. Early in practice, predictable routines may increase the anticipation of sensory stimuli and reduce reaction time.
The ultimate goal for variable practice is to transfer to the natural environment. To **enhance** transfer to the natural environment, teach the child to attend to salient features of the environment. Also progress toward automatic performance of the motor task to enhance transfer to novel conditions. Test for automatic performance by presenting competing tasks during practice and observing their effects on performance.	Practice in the natural environment may be affected by limited **information processing** resources and **reduced automatic performance**. Some clinical populations demonstrate a decrement in performance of a postural control task when given a concurrent cognitive task, which competes with attention (Huang & Mercer, 2001). Limitations with automaticity could affect performance under novel conditions, where attention resources are directed toward exploring the features of the environment and task.

tice of the stair task, physical guidance provided during the trial, and feedback provided after the trial. According to motor learning principles, instruction focuses attention to the task requirements and sets goals for the performer. Instructions should be brief and simple, and direct focus onto the relevant cues of the task (Schmidt & Wrisberg, 2000). They should focus attention onto the external aspects of performance (Wulf, Hoess, & Prinz, 1998), not the movement itself. These recommendations seem to be directly applicable to instruction for children. They may be enhanced by the adaptations presented in Table 2. For Clara, focus would be on the stair riser rather than flexion of her legs.

TABLE 2. Proposed Adaptations to Instruction and Related Special Learning Needs

Proposed Adaptations to Instruction	Special Learning Need Related to Motor Learning Mechanism
Enhance verbal demonstrations by cueing the child to the relevant issues of the task. When presenting a task, allow time for processing the information. Demonstration may be more beneficial than verbal cues for some children.	Children with neurological conditions may require increased time for **information processing.**

Feedback is provided to help evaluate performance and detect errors. Knowledge of results is augmented information provided after the action is completed to indicate how the performer achieved the desired outcome of the action (Schmidt & Wrisberg, 2000). Knowledge of performance, which is feedback about movement patterns used to perform the action, is recommended for complex functional skills (Schmidt & Wrisberg, 2000). In adults, there is strong evidence that "less feedback is better." According to the guidance principle, too much information may cause a dependency and diminish active processing necessary for encoding into long-term memory (Winstein, 1991). There are developmental factors related to the time required to process feedback and the precision of information that can be processed (Newell & Kennedy, 1978; Newell & Carlton, 1980; Gallagher & Thomas, 1979). Proposed adaptations to augmented information, which should be examined empirically, are presented in Table 3.

Impairment-Focused Interventions

Meeting the individual needs of the child may require integration of impairment-level intervention and activity-focused intervention. According to Campbell (1991) and Heriza and Sweeney (1994), problem solving about impairments begins after the specified functional goals are established. Impairment-level interventions may be indicated, not only to support function, but also to reduce the risk of secondary disability. Impairments comprise personal constraints that determine which task and environment interventions will be effective. Impairments associated with neurological conditions are numerous and have a unique expression in each child. Likewise, the interventions are numerous and should be individualized. According to Figure 1, impairment-focused intervention can be systematically integrated with the activity-focused intervention.

TABLE 3. Proposed Adaptations to Augmented Information and Related Special Learning Needs

Proposed Adaptations to Practice	Special Learning Need Related to Motor Learning Mechanism
Modify the frequency and amount of feedback to meet individual needs.	Guidelines for amount and frequency of feedback and other forms of augmented information assume intact **error detection**. Error detection capabilities may be impaired in children with neurological conditions, due to impairments in sensory functions and increased inter-trial variability. Impairments in motor control may increase the complexity of the motor challenge for children with neurological conditions and prolong the early phase of practice, which has increased requirement for augmented information.
Modify the type of augmented information. Knowledge of results may be redundant with practical tasks. The outcome of a practice trial (e.g., ascending a step) is naturally evident to the child. Furthermore, given the attention and information processing requirements, knowledge of performance may not be suitable for children with neurological disorders. Transition information, which guides the child on how to improve future performance, based on previous performance, may be more useful (Kernodle & Carlton, 1992) than feedback. The role of the change agent is to support the search for the coordination that will meet task demands. Use physical guidance early in practice to provide the "feel of the movement." Physical guidance may accelerate the early phases of learning and help the child to develop a basic plan of action. The child can then engage in active problem solving to meet task requirements.	Challenges with **information processing** mechanisms challenge automatic performance. If **automatic performance** is not achieved, attention resources must be allocated to performance of even basic movements. This limits attention resources for processing complicated kinematic information provided in knowledge of performance. Children with neurological conditions often have difficulty developing or retrieving a plan of action because of limitations in **feedforward modes of control**.

Impairment-Focused Interventions Which Involve Functional Activity

Active impairment-level interventions involve purposeful activity. Because motor control and coordination emerge in the context of purposeful activity, impairments should, ideally, be ameliorated through practice of meaningful functional tasks. Impairments that limit the performance of critical components of movement may be ameliorated through process of improving the child's ability to adapt motor behavior to meet task demands. For example, Clara's difficulty with the foot placement on the step may relate to impairments in force production, selective control of leg flexion, and postural control. Active practice addresses these impairments with the context of the task.

When impairment is addressed through functional activity, augmented information and other practice strategies might enhance learning. In addition, therapeutic procedures, which address impairments in the context of activity, may enhance motor learning. One example is the use of neuromuscular electrical stimulation during practice of gait or upper extremity activities (Carmick, 1995, 1997). The sensory cues as well as the stimulation of muscle provide input that should enhance active movement. Facilitation and inhibition techniques that address patterns of movement, early in practice (Bly, 1991), might be considered impairment-related enhancements. However, they do not enhance learning if they limit active exploration.

Therapeutic enhancements of practice also include task or environmental manipulations such as a treadmill surface to induce coordination of stepping, (Schindl, Forstner, Kern, & Hesse, 2000) or a water medium, which permits use of buoyancy or resistance of the water medium (Dumas & Francesconi, 2000). Hippotherapy and therapeutic riding address impaired posture, balance and mobility (MacKinnon, Noh, Laliberte, Laliviere, & Allan, 1995; McGibbon, Andrade, Widener, & Cintas, 1998).

Impairment-Focused Interventions Which Involve Therapeutic Activity

The other category of active impairment-level interventions primarily focuses on therapeutic activities intended to reduce impairments, rather than purposeful activity. Resistive exercise with free weights or an isokinetic device is an example. Research evidence supports the use of resistive exercise for increasing strength in children with cerebral palsy (Damiano & Able, 1998; Damiano, Dodd, & Taylor, 2002; Darrah, Fan, Chen, Nunweiler, & Watkins, 1997).

Passive Impairment-Focused Interventions

Passive procedures do not require participation in purposeful activity by the child. Passive procedures include: (1) procedures directed toward the impairment, not administered in the context of a purposeful task or activity, and (2) passive procedures that are preparatory to a purposeful task or activity. Passive procedures not administered in context of purposeful activities are usually interventions directed toward reducing secondary impairments of joint limitations or soft tissue contractures associated with muscle tone disorders. Therapeutic electrical stimulation administered to children during sleeping hours is an example (Dali et al., 2000). Clara sits in a long-sitter for thirty minutes and has maintained length in hamstrings after surgery.

The second category includes preparatory procedures performed by the therapist to create a more optimal readiness of certain systems, mostly the musculolskeletal system, prior to a motor learning experience. Procedures to reduce soft tissue problems associated with spasticity are often used by physical and occupational therapists as preparatory to practice (Boehme, 1988; Kluzik, Fetters, & Coryell, 1990). Clara has a pelvic asymmetry due to compensations for pelvic instability and muscle tone imbalance. Prior to practice on the steps, her physical therapist might elongate soft tissue structures and reduce over activity in certain muscle groups. Also elongation of the heel cord helps to place the foot more optimally in the hinged-ankle-foot orthosis making it easier for the tibia to move over the foot while ascending the stairs.

The need for and effectiveness of these preparatory techniques must be evaluated for each child and a topic for clinical research. According to current models of intervention, therapists should not create a long-term dependence on these passive procedures. The important question is: Will the child be able to perform the task in the real environment when the passive procedures are not available? The ability of the child, over time, to perform his or her own preparatory activity should be considered.

CONCLUSION

The proposed practice model describes the role of the physical therapist and occupational therapist as a change agent in activity-focused interventions for children with neurological conditions. The model integrates impairment-focused intervention with activity-focused intervention. Emphasis is placed on functional activity and adapting motor learning processes based on the child's individual strengths and learning challenges. There is a need for research to determine optimal guidelines for motor learning of functional activities and adaptations to them for children with neurological conditions.

REFERENCES

Bartlett, D. J. & Palisano, R. J. (2002). Physical therapists' perceptions of factors influencing the acquisition of motor abilities of children with cerebral palsy: Implications for clinical reasoning. *Physical Therapy, 82*, 237-248.

Bernstein, N. (1967). *The co-ordination and regulation of movements.* New York: Pergamon.

Blanche, E. I. & Nakasuji, B. (2000). Sensory integration and the child with cerebral palsy. In S. Roley, E. I. Blanche & R. C. Shaaf (Eds.), *Understanding the nature of sensory integration with diverse populations*, pp. 345-364. Therapy Skill Builders.

Bly, L. (1991). A historical and current view of the basis of NDT. *Pediatric Physical Therapy*, 3 (3), 131-135.

Bly, L. (1996). What is the role of sensation in motor learning? What is the role of feedback and feedforward? *Neurodevelopmental Treatment Association Network, 5* (5), 1-7.

Boehme, R. (1988). *Improving upper body control.* San Antonio, TX: Therapy Skill Builders.

Campbell, P. H. (1991). Evaluation and assessment in early intervention for infants and toddlers. *Journal of Early Interventions, 15* (42), 36-45.

Carmick, J. (1995). Managing equinus in children with cerebral palsy: Electrical stimulation to the triceps surae muscle. *Developmental Medicine and Child Neurology, 37*, 965-975.

Carmick, J. (1997). Use of neuromuscular electrical stimulation and dorsal wrist splint to improve the hand function of a child with spastic hemiparesis. *Physical Therapy, 77*, 661-671.

Carson, L. M. & Wigand, R. L. (1979). Motor schema formation and retention in young children: A test of Schmidt's schema theory. *Journal of Motor Behavior, 11*, 247-251.

Christina, R. W. (1982). Simple reaction time as a function of response complexity: Memory drum theory revisited. *Journal of Motor Behavior, 14*, 301-321.

Clark, J. E. (1995). Dynamic systems perspective on gait. In R. L. Craik & C. A. Oatis (Eds.), *Gait Analysis: Theory and Application* (pp. 79-86). St. Louis: Mosby.

Clark, J. E. (1997). A dynamical systems perspective on the development of complex adaptive skill. In C. Dent-Read & P. Zukow-Goldring (Eds.), *Evolving explanations of development* (pp. 383-406). Washington, DC: American Psychological Association.

Dali, C., Hansen, F. J., Pedersen, S. A., Skov, L., Hilden, J., Bjornskov, L., Strandberg, C., Jette, C., Ulla, H., Herbst, G. & Ulla, L. (2002). Threshold electrical stimulation in ambulant children with CP: A randomized double-blind placebo-controlled clinical trial. *Developmental Medicine & Child Neurology, 44*, 364-369.

Damiano, D. L. & Able, M. F. (1998). Functional outcomes of strength training in spastic cerebral palsy. *Archives of Physical Medicine and Rehabilitation, 79*, 119-125.

Damiano, D. L., Dodd, K. & Taylor, N. F. (2002). Should we be testing and training muscle strength in cerebral palsy? *Developmental Medicine and Child Neurology, 44*, 68-72.

Darrah, J., Fan, J. S., Chen, L., Nunweiler, J. & Watkins, B. (1997). Review of the effects of progressive resistive muscle strengthening in children with cerebral palsy: A clinical consensus. *Pediatric Physical Therapy, 9*,12-17.

Darrah, J. & Bartlett, D. (1995). Dynamic systems theory and management of children with cerebral palsy: Unresolved issues. *Infants and Young Chilren, 8*, 52-59.

Duff, S. & Quinn, L. (2000). Motor learning and motor control. In D. Cech & S. Martin (Eds.) *Functional movement development across the life span, 2nd Edition* (pp. 86-117). Philadelphia, PA: W.B. Saunders.

Dumas, H. & Francesconi, S. (2002). Aquatic therapy in paediatrics: Annotated bibliography. *Physical & Occupational Therapy in Pediatrics, 20*, 63-78.

Eliasson, A. C., Gordon, A. M. & Forssberg, H. (1991). Basic co-ordination of manipulative forces in children with cerebral palsy. *Developmental Medicine and Child Neurology, 33*, 661-170.

Eliasson, A. C., Gordon, A.M., & Forssberg, H. (1992). Impaired anticipatory control of isometric forces during grasping by children with cerebral palsy. *Developmental Medicine and Child Neurology, 34*, 216-225.

Eliasson, A. C., Gordon, A. M., & Forssberg, H. (1995). Tactile control of isometric forces during grasping in children with cerebral palsy. *Developmental Medicine and Child Neurology, 37*, 72-84.

Gage, J. (1991). *Gait analysis in cerebral palsy*. New York, NY: Cambridge University Press.

Gallagher, J. & Thomas, J.R. (1980). Effects of varying post-KR intervals upon children's performance. *Journal of Motor Behavior, 12*, 41-46.

Gentile, A.M. (1992). The nature of skill acquisition: Therapeutic implications for children with movement disorders. In H. Forssberg & H. Hirschfeld (Eds.), *Movement disorders in children. Medical Sport Science*, vol. 36 (pp. 31-40). Basel: Karger.

Goodgold-Edwards, S. A. & Gianutsis, J. G. (1991). Coincidence anticipation performance of children with spastic cerebral palsy and non-handicapped children. *Physical & Occupational Therapy in Pediatrics, 10*, 49-82.

Gordon, A. M. & Duff, S. V. (1999). Fingertip forces during object manipulation in children with hemiplegic cerebral palsy: Anticipatory scaling. *Developmental Medicine and Child Neurology, 41*, 166-175.

Guide to Physical Therapist Practice (1999). Alexandria, VA: American Physical Therapy Association.

Hadders-Algra, M. (2000). The neuronal group selection theory: Promising principles for understanding and treating developmental motor disorders. *Developmental Medicine and Child Neurology, 42*, 707-715.

Haken, H., Kelso, J. A. S. & Bunz, H. (1985). A theoretical model of phase transitions in human hand movements. *Biological Cybernetics, 39*, 139-56.

Harbourne, R. T. (2001). Accuracy of movement speed and error detection skills in adolescents with cerebral palsy. *Perceptual and Motor Skills, 93*, 419-431.

Hayes, M. S., McEwen, I. R, Lovett, D., Sheldon, M. M. & Smith, D. (1999). Next Step: Survey of pediatric physical therapists' educational needs and perceptions of motor control, motor development and motor learning as they relate to services for children with developmental disabilities. *Pediatric Physical Therapy, 11*, 164-182.

Heriza, C.B. (1991). Motor development: Traditional and contemporary theories. In: Lister, M.J. (Ed.), *Contemporary management of motor problems: Proceedings of the II Step Conference* (pp. 99-126). Alexandria, VA: American Physical Therapy Association.

Heriza, C. B. & Sweeney, J. K. (1994). Pediatric physical therapy: Part 1. Practice, scope, scientific basis, and theoretical foundation. *Infants and Young Children, 7,* 20-32.

Horak, F.B. (1991). Assumptions underlying motor control for neurologic rehabilitation. In J. J. Lister (Ed.) *Contemporary management of motor control problems* (pp. 11-28). Alexandria, VA: American Physical Therapy Association.

Horne, E. M., Warren, S. F. & Jones, H. A. (1995). An experimental analysis of a neurobehavioral motor intervention. *Developmental Medicine and Child Neurology, 37,* 697-714.

Howard, E. M. & Henderson, S. E. (1989). Perceptual problems in cerebral-palsied children: A real-world example. *Human Movement Science, 8,* 141-160.

Huang, H. & Mercer, V. (2001). Dual task methodology: Application in studies of cognitive and motor performance in adults and children. *Pediatric Physical Therapy, 13,* 133-140.

Huang, H., Mercer, V. & Thorpe, D. (2003). Effects of different concurrent cognitive tasks on temporal-distance gait variables in children. *Pediatric Physical Therapy, 15,* 105-113.

International Classification of Functioning, Disability and Health (ICF) (2001). World Health Organization.

Kelso, J. A. S. (1984). Phase transitions and critical behavior in human bimanual coordination. *American Journal of Physiology. 15,* R10000-R10004.

Kernodle, M. W. & Carlton, L. G. (1992). Information feedback and the learning of multiple-degree of freedom activities. *Journal of Motor Behaviour, 24,* 187-196.

Ketelaar, M., Vermer, A., Hart, H., van Petegem-van Beek, E. & Helders, P. J. (2001). Effects of a functional therapeutic program on motor abilities of children with cerebral palsy. *Physical Therapy, 8,* 1534-1545.

King, E. M., Gooch, J. L, Howell, G. H., Peters, M. L., Bloswick, D. S. & Brown, D. R. (1993). Evaluation of the hip-extensor tricycle in improving gait in children with cerebral palsy. *Developmental Medicine and Child Neurology, 35,* 1048-54.

Larin, H. (2000). Motor learning: Theories and strategies for the practitioner. In S. K. Campbell (Ed.), *Physical therapy for children, 2nd edition.* (pp. 170-195). Philadelphia, PA: W.B. Saunders Co.

Lee, D. N. & Cook, M. L. (1990). Basic perceptuo-motor dysfunctions in cerebral palsy. In J. Jeannerod (Ed.), *Attention and performance XIII: Motor representation and control* (pp. 583-602). New Jersey: Laurence Erlbaum Associates, Publishers.

Lesny, I., Nachtmann, M., Stehlik, A., Tomankova, A. & Zajdkova, J. (1990). Disorders of memory of motor sequences in cerebral palsied children. *Brain and Development, 12,* 339-41.

Light, K. E. (1991). Issues of cognition for motor control. In P.C. Montgomery & B. H. Connolly (Eds.), *Motor control and physical therapy: Theoretical framework and practical application* (pp. 85-98). Hixson, TN: Chattanooga Group, Inc.

Mac Kinnon, J. R., Noh, S., Laliberte, D., Lariviere, J. & Allan, D. E. (1995). Therapeutic horseback riding: A review of the literature. *Physical & Occupational Therapy in Pediatrics,* 15, 1-15.

McEwen, I. R. (2000). Children with cognitive impairments. In S. K. Campbell, D. W. Vander Linden & J. Palisano (Eds.) *Physical Therapy for Children* (2nd ed., pp. 502-531). Philadelphia: W.B. Saunders.

McEwen, I. & Shelden, M. L. (1995). Pediatric therapy in the 1990's: The demise of educational versus medical dichotomy. *Physical & Occupational Therapy in Pediatrics, 15,* 33-45.

McGibbon, H., Andrade, C., Widener, G. & Cintas, H. L. (1998). Effect of an equine-movement therapy program on gait, energy expenditure, and motor function in children with spastic cerebral palsy: A pilot study. *Developmental Medicine and Child Neurology, 40,* 754-762.

Newell, K.M. (1986). Constraints on the development of co-ordination. In M.G. Wade & H. T. A. Whiting (Eds.), Motor development in children: Aspects of co-ordination and control. Boston, MA: Martinus Nyhoff.

Newell, K. M. (1996). Change in movement and skill: Learning, retention, and transfer. In: M. Latash, M. T. Turvey (Eds.) *Dexterity and its development* (pp. 339-376). Mahwah, NJ: Lawrence Erlbaum Associates.

Newell, K. M. & Carlton, L. G. (1980). Developmental trends in motor response recognition. *Developmental Psychology, 16,* 550-554.

Newell, K. M. & Kennedy, J. A. Knowledge of results and children's motor learning. *Developmental Psychobiology, 14,* 531-536.

Newell, K. M., Morris, L. R. & Scully, D. M. (1990). Augmented information and the acquisition of skill in physical activity. In R. L. Terjung (Ed.) *Exercise and Sport Science Reviews,* 235-262.

Newell, K. M. & Valvano, J. (1998). Therapeutic intevention as a constraint in the learning and relearning of movement skills. *Scandinavian Journal of Occupational Therapy, 5,* 51-57.

Olney, S. J. & Wright, M. J. (2000). Cerebral palsy. In S. K. Campbell (Ed.) *Physical therapy for children, 2nd edition.* (pp. 533-570). Philadelphia, PA: W. B. Saunders Co.

Palisano, R., Rosenbaum, P., Walter, S., Russell, D., Wood, E. & Galuppi, B. (1997). Development and reliability of a system to classify gross motor function in children with cerebral palsy. *Developmental Medicine and Child Neurology, 39,* 214-223.

Parks, S., Rose, D. J., & Dunn, J. M. (1989) A comparison of fractionated reaction time between cerebral palsied and non-handicapped youths. *Adapted Physical Activity Quarterly, 6,* 379-388.

Schindl, M. R., Forstner, C., Kern, H. & Hesse, S. (2000). Treadmill training with partial body weight support in nonambulatory patients with cerebral palsy. *Archives of Physical Medicine and Rehabilitation, 81,* 301-306.

Scholz, J. P. (1990). Dynamic pattern theory—some implications for therapeutics. *Physical Therapy, 70,* 827-843.

Scholz, J. P. & Kelso, J. A. S. (1990). Intentional switching between patterns of bimanual coordination depends on the intrinsic dynamics of the patterns. *Journal of Motor Behavior, 22,* 98-124.

Schmidt, R. A. & Wrisberg, C. A. (2000). *Motor Performance and Learning*. Champaign, IL: Human Kinetics.

Schmidt, R. A. (1988). *Motor control and learning: A behavioural emphasis* (2nd ed.). Champaign: IL: Human Kinetics Publishers.

Scolz, J. P. & Kelso, J. A. S. (1990). A quantitative approach to understanding the formation and change of coordinated movement patterns. *Journal of Motor Behavior, 21,* 122-144.

Smethust, C. J. & Carson, R. G. (2003). The effect of volition on the stability of bimanual coordination. *Journal of Motor Behavior, 35,* 309-319.

Stiers, P., Vanderkelen, R., Vanneste, G., Coene, S., De Rammeleraere, M. & Vandenbussche, E. (2002). Visual-perceptual impairment in a random sample of children with cerebral palsy. *Developmental Medicine and Child Neurology, 44,* 370-382.

Sugden, D. A. & Keogh, J. F. (1990). *Problems in Movement Skill Development*. Columbia, SC: University of South Carolina Press.

Thelan, E. (1986). Development of coordinated movement: Implications for early hyman development. In H. T. A. Whiting (Ed.) *Motor development in children: Aspects of coordination and control* (pp. 107-120). Boston: Martinus Nijhoff.

Thorpe, D. E. & Valvano, J. (2002). The effects of knowledge of results and cognitive strategies on motor skill learning by children with cerebral palsy. *Pediatric Physical Therapy, 14,* 2-15.

Valvano, J., Heriza, C. B. & Carollo, J. (2003). The effects of physical and verbal guidance on the learning of a gross motor skill by children with cerebral palsy. Unpublished data.

Valvano, J. & Newell, K. M. (1998). Practice of a precision isometric grip force task by children with spastic cerebral palsy. *Developmental Medicine and Child Neurology, 40,* 464-473.

Valvano, J., Westcott, S. & Palisano, R. J. (1998). Quantifying change over practice by children with spastic cerebral palsy. *Pediatric Physical Therapy, 10,* 184.

Van der Weel, van der Meer, A. & Lee, D. (1991). Effect of task on movement control in cerebral palsy: Implications for assessment and therapy. *Developmental Medicine and Child Neurology, 33,* 419-426.

Wenderoth, N., Bock, O. & Krohn, R. (2002). Learning a new bimanual coordination pattern is influenced by existing attractors. *Motor Control, 6,* 166-182.

Winstein, C. J. (1991). Designing practice for motor learning: Clinical implications. In: Lister, M. J. (Ed.) *Contemporary management of motor problems: Proceedings of the II Step Conference* (pp. 65-76). Alexandria, VA: American Physical Therapy Association.

Winstein, C. J., Gardner, E. R., McNeal, D. R., Barto, P. S. & Nicholson, D. E. (1989). Standing balance training: Effects on balance and locomotion in hemiparetic adults. *Archives of Physical Medicine and Rehabilitation, 70,* 755-762.

Wulf, G. (1991). The effect of practice on motor learning in children. *Applied Cognitive Psychology, 5:* 123-134.

Wulf, G., Hoess, M. & Prinz, W. (1998). Instructions for motor learning: Differential effects of internal versus external focus of attention. *Journal of Motor Behavior, 30,* 169-179.

Yao, M. (1995). *Patterns of prehension in young children with cerebral palsy.* Unpublished masters thesis.

Zanone, P. & Kelso, J. A. S. (1991). Experimental studies of behavioral attractors and their evolution with learning. In. J. Requin & G. E. Stelmach (Eds.), *Tutorals in motor neuroscience* (pp. 121-133). Netherlands: Kluwer Academic Publishers.

Zanone, P. G. & Kelso, J. A. S. (1994). The coordination dynamics of learning: Theoretical structure and research agenda. In S. Swinnen, H. Heuer, J. Massion & P. Casaer (Eds.), *Inter-limb coordination* (pp. 461-490). San Diego, CA: Academic Press.

Zanone, P. G., Kelso, J. A. S. & Jeka, J. J. (1993). Concepts and methods for a dynamical approach to behavioral coordination and change. In G. J. P. Savelsbergh (Ed.), *The development of coordination in infancy* (pp. 89-153). Elsevier Science Publishers.

Changes in Mobility of Children
with Cerebral Palsy Over Time
and Across Environmental Settings

Beth L. Tieman
Robert J. Palisano
Edward J. Gracely
Peter L. Rosenbaum
Lisa A. Chiarello
Margaret E. O'Neil

Beth L. Tieman, PT, PhD, is Assistant Professor, Department of Physical Therapy, Georgia State University, Atlanta, GA. Robert J. Palisano, PT, ScD, is Professor, Programs in Rehabilitation Sciences, Drexel University, Philadelphia, PA. Edward J. Gracely, PhD, is Associate Professor, Department of Family, Community, and Preventive Medicine, Drexel University, Philadelphia, PA. Peter L. Rosenbaum, MD, FRCP(C), is Professor of Paediatrics, McMaster University, Co-Director, CanChild Centre for Childhood Disability Research, and Canada Research Chair in Childhood Disability, Ontario, Canada. Lisa A. Chiarello, PT, PhD, PCS, is Associate Professor, Programs in Rehabilitation Sciences, Drexel University, Philadelphia, PA. Margaret E. O'Neil, PT, PhD, MPH, is Assistant Professor, Programs in Rehabilitation Sciences, Drexel University, Philadelphia, PA.

This work was supported by grant MCJ429391 from the Department of Health and Human Services, Maternal and Child Health Bureau, awarded to Drexel University; grant MT-13476 from the Canadian Institutes of Health Research (formerly the Medical Research Council of Canada); and grant RO1-HD-34947 from the National Center for Medical Rehabilitation Research of the National Institute of Child Health and Human Development.

[Haworth co-indexing entry note]: "Changes in Mobility of Children with Cerebral Palsy Over Time and Across Environmental Settings." Tieman et al. Co-published simultaneously in *Physical & Occupational Therapy in Pediatrics* (The Haworth Press, Inc.) Vol. 24, No. 1/2, 2004, pp. 109-128; and: *Movement Sciences: Transfer of Knowledge into Pediatric Therapy Practice* (ed: Robert J. Palisano) The Haworth Press, Inc., 2004, pp. 109-128. Single or multiple copies of this article are available for a fee from The Haworth Document Delivery Service [1-800-HAWORTH, 9:00 a.m. - 5:00 p.m. (EST). E-mail address: docdelivery@haworthpress.com].

SUMMARY. This study examined changes in mobility methods of children with cerebral palsy (CP) over time and across environmental settings. Sixty-two children with CP, ages 6-14 years and classified as levels II-IV on the Gross Motor Function Classification System, were randomly selected from a larger data base and followed for three to four years. On each of several assessments, parents completed a questionnaire on their child's usual mobility methods in the home, school, and outdoors/community settings. During the first assessment interval, mobility methods increased to methods requiring more gross motor control. During the second assessment interval, mobility methods were unchanged or decreased to methods requiring less gross motor control. Changes within the child and within the environment are hypothesized to occur and to impact changes in mobility methods. Screening at regular intervals is recommended to monitor changes in mobility. Interventions to enhance mobility may be indicated during periods of change in the child or exposure to new environments. *[Article copies available for a fee from The Haworth Document Delivery Service: 1-800-HAWORTH. E-mail address: <docdelivery@haworthpress.com> Website: <http://www.HaworthPress. com> © 2004 by The Haworth Press, Inc. All rights reserved.]*

KEYWORDS. Mobility, cerebral palsy, environmental setting, longitudinal

Cerebral palsy (CP) refers to a non-progressive insult to the central nervous system (Bax, 1964), but the impairments associated with CP continue to change throughout an individual's lifespan (Mutch, Alberman, Hagberg, Kodama, & Perat, 1992). During middle childhood and early adolescence, changes in body structure and function, and the contextual features of environmental settings, may all affect mobility. Because mobility is important for the performance of many activities (e.g., self-care and social activities), changes in mobility may affect overall participation in society, including access to education, the community, and future employment (Pollock & Stewart, 1990; Modell, Rider, & Menchetti, 1997).

Previous research has examined differences in mobility of children with CP across environmental setting (Haley, Coster, & Binder-Sundberg, 1994; Berry, McLaurin, & Sparling, 1996; Pollock & Stewart, 1998; Tieman, 2002; Palisano et al., 2003). These studies provide some quantitative evidence that mobility methods vary across environmental setting (Tieman, 2002), specifically in terms of use of battery-powered wheelchairs (Berry et al., 1996), and degree of adult assistance (Haley et al., 1994; Palisano et al., 2003). For instance, children use independent mobility methods more at home than at school and dependent methods more in the outdoors/community than at school (Palisano et al., 2003). While these studies provide evidence of the influence of environmental setting on mobility in children with CP, changes in mobility over time have not previously been examined. Longitudinal research on mobility in children with CP is limited to studies focusing on the prediction of independent ambulation using motor milestones (Bottos et al., 1989; Campos da Paz, Burnett, & Braga, 1994; Trahan & Marcoux, 1994; Bottos, Puato, Vianello, & Facchin, 1995; Scrutton & Rosenbaum, 1997; Montgomery, 1998). There has been no research to examine how other mobility methods (e.g., walking with a walking aid, using battery-powered wheelchair) used by children with CP change over time across different settings.

The concept of person-environment interaction illustrated in Figure 1 provides a framework for understanding the performance of mobility in children with CP. Simeonsson, Lollar, Hollowell, and Adams (2000) stated that the relationship between the child and environment is dynamic, reciprocal, and changes over time. The construct "person" includes both capability (e.g., gross motor, fine motor, and cognitive development) and personal factors (e.g., personality, habits, interests, motivation and lifestyle) (WHO, 2001). Capability (sometimes referred to as "capacity") is defined as the child's abilities, or what a child can do in a controlled environment (Young, Williams, Yoshida, Bombadier, & Wright, 1996; WHO, 2001). Capability may be influenced by age-related changes such as physical growth (e.g., musculoskeletal changes, weight gain, and neurological maturation), social expectations, and cognition. Changes in personal factors, such as a child's comfort with a mobility aid and motivation to keep up with peers, also may affect method of mobility (Law et al., 1998).

The construct "environment" includes contextual features, the physical, temporal, and social features of everyday settings of home, school, outdoors, and community that may change over time. Physical and temporal demands may change such that children are required to move longer distances and at faster speeds in order to keep up with peers. Social features are especially important in settings where peer interaction is present, such as the school, outdoors, and community. Children may adapt performance of mobility to accommodate to these changes in contextual features of the environment.

FIGURE 1. Person-environment interaction in the performance of mobility. Changes over time may occur in the person, environment, and the person-environment interaction, thereby influencing the performance of mobility.

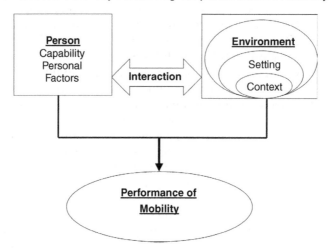

The purpose of this study was to examine changes over time and across settings in the usual mobility methods of children with CP, ages 6-14 years, classified at levels II-IV on the Gross Motor Function Classification System (GMFCS) (Palisano et al., 1997). The research questions were: (1) Do mobility methods change over a 3-4 year period? and (2) Do changes in mobility methods differ across the home, school, and outdoors/community settings?

METHOD

Subjects

Sixty-two children were included in this study. The subjects were selected from a larger pool of children who participated in a longitudinal study of the development of gross motor function (Rosenbaum et al., 2002). Subjects in the longitudinal study were randomly selected from 19 of the 20 centers providing children's rehabilitation services throughout Ontario. The 19 centers identified 2108 children with CP who met the criteria for inclusion in the longitudinal study. From this population, a sample of 1304 children was randomly selected and stratified by age and

Gross Motor Function Classification System (GMFCS) level (Palisano et al., 1997). Three hundred sixty-six children were ineligible or unavailable for various reasons. Of the remaining 938 children, 721 families (77%) agreed to participate and 682 children provided at least one observation for the longitudinal study. The 682 children in the longitudinal study ranged in age from 1-14 years at the start of the study and either had a diagnosis of cerebral palsy made by a physician or had motor impairments consistent with CP. The definition of CP proposed by Bax (1964) was used. None of the children had received selective dorsal rhizotomy surgery, intrathecal baclofen, or botulinum toxin injections in the lower limbs prior to study recruitment, because these interventions potentially alter gross motor function. None of these interventions was readily available in Ontario at the time of the study.

Of the 682 children in the longitudinal study, 391 children were between 6 and 14 years of age, had a diagnosis of CP, and had completed the final assessment of the longitudinal study, corresponding to Time 3 of this study (Table 1). Of these 391 children, 124 children had completed parent questionnaires at all assessments of the longitudinal study. Sixty-three of these children were classified at GMFCS levels II-IV. The decision to include in this study only children classified at levels II, III, and IV was made because these children tend to demonstrate more variability in mobility methods than children at levels I and V (Palisano et al., 2003). The age range of 6 to 14 years was selected, as there is evidence indicating that gross motor capability of children with CP begins to plateau at an average age of 2.7 to 4.8 years of age depending on gross motor classification level (Rosenbaum et al., 2002). One child was eliminated from this study because the parent had not completed the questionnaire clearly, so the final number of children used in data analysis for this study was N = 62.

The mean age of children at the first assessment was 8.3 years (Table 2). At the second and third assessments, the mean ages were 10.4 years and

TABLE 1. Sampling Frame from Longitudinal Study

N = 682	Children ages 1-14 years who completed the first assessment in the longitudinal study
N = 391	Children ages 6-14 years who completed the final assessment
N = 124	Children who had completed parent questionnaires at all assessments
N = 63	Children classified at GMFCS Levels II - IV at all assessments
N = 62	Final number of children used in data analysis (after one parent questionnaire excluded)

TABLE 2. Ages of Children at Each Assessment Period

	Time 1	Time 2	Time 3
Age range	6 - 10 years	7 - 13 years	9 - 14 years
Mean (SD)	8.3 years (1.5)	10.4 years (1.5)	12.1 years (1.4)

12.1 years, respectively. The sample consisted of 32 boys (52%) and 30 girls (48%). At the first assessment, there were 11 (18%) children classified at level II, 30 (48%) at level III, and 21 (34%) at level IV of the GMFCS. The proportion of children at each GMFCS level remained relatively stable throughout the course of the study, consistent with a previous study of the test-retest reliability of the GMFCS (Wood & Rosenbaum, 2000).

Measures

Gross Motor Function Classification System

The GMFCS is a five-level system used to classify a child's level of gross motor function, based on usual performance in home, school, and outdoors/community settings (Palisano et al., 1997). By age 6, children in level II walk without assistive devices but have limitations walking outdoors and in the community. Children in level III walk with assistive mobility devices but have limitations walking outdoors and in the community. Children in level IV have self-mobility (e.g., power mobility) with limitations and are transported or use power mobility outdoors and in the community. There is evidence of the validity and reliability, including test-retest reliability and interrater reliability of the GMFCS (Palisano et al., 1997; Palisano et al., 2000; Wood & Rosenbaum, 2000; Rosenbaum et al., 2002). The use of the GMFCS requires familiarity with the child, but no formal training.

In this study, GMFCS levels were determined at the first assessment by 36 physical therapists who had an average of 12.2 years experience (SD = 7.2), ranging from 1 year to 32 years experience. The therapist who determined the GMFCS level did not necessarily provide services to the child. The therapist also administered the Gross Motor Function Measure (GMFM) (Russell, Rosenbaum, Avery, & Lane, 2002), data from which are not presented in this study.

Parent Questionnaire

A parent questionnaire, developed specifically for the longitudinal study, included information pertaining to the child's usual mobility methods in the home, school, and outdoors/community settings. Several authors support using parent report to measure the performance of children in everyday settings. Long (1992) stated that parent report is appropriate when measuring the typical performance of children, in order to consider performance across various settings. In support of this idea, Wilson, Kaplan, Crawford, Campbell, and Dewey (2000) stated that parent questionnaires provide a qualitative, accurate assessment of their children's skills in a naturalistic environment. Parent report of children's current skills has consistently been shown to be a sensitive, reliable and valid source of information (Wilson et al., 2000). The questionnaire in this study utilized a recognition format (Does your child use *walking alone* in the home?) that has greater reliability than an identification format (What mobility method does your child use at home?) (Glascoe & Dworkin, 1995).

The questionnaire instructed parents to choose the *one* mobility method that best describes the child's "usual way of getting around" in each of the following settings: (1) home, (2) school, and (3) outdoors or in the community. For each setting, parents had to choose *one* of the following mobility methods: (a) carried by an adult, (b) pushed by an adult in a stroller, wheelchair, or other similar piece of equipment, (c) rolls, creeps, or crawls on the floor, (d) takes steps holding onto walls or furniture, (e) takes steps holding onto an adult's hands, (f) walks using a walking aid (a piece of equipment), (g) walks alone without any assistance, (h) propels self in regular wheelchair, (i) operates a battery wheelchair, or (j) not applicable.

Procedure

The parent questionnaire, GMFCS, and Gross Motor Function Measure (GMFM) (Russell et al., 1993) were administered at five points in the longitudinal study. For this study, data from three time points (Time 1, Time 2, and Time 3) were analyzed. Table 3 reports the time intervals (in years) between the assessments. Children were followed for a total length ranging from 3 years to 4.4 years.

At the first assessment, the parent questionnaire was completed by the child's mother (N = 53, 85%), father (N = 7, 11%), or both parents (N = 2, 3%). Only those assessments completed by parents, and not

TABLE 3. Time Intervals Between Assessment Periods

	First time interval Time 1 to Time 2	Second time interval Time 2 to Time 3	Total study time Time 1 to Time 3
Age (minimum-maximum)	1.6 - 2.5 years	1.3 - 2.3 years	3 - 4.4 years
Mean (SD)	2.0 years (.18)	1.7 years (.23)	3.7 years (.31)

other caregivers, were included in data analysis, but it is unknown if the same parent completed all of the questionnaires throughout the study. Although parents were instructed to choose one method when reporting their children's usual mobility, one parent reported more than one method in the school setting, and therefore data for this child were excluded from analysis.

Data Analysis

In order to analyze differences in mobility across settings, the nine mobility methods from the parent questionnaire were converted from nominal level data into ordinal level data using a ranking system (Table 4). The ranking system was created using empirical data and was based on the construct of the trunk and lower extremity *motor control required to perform each mobility method.* The highest ranked method (1), walking alone, reflects the most trunk and lower extremity motor control requirements, whereas the lowest rank method (9), being pushed by an adult, reflects the least trunk and lower extremity motor control requirements for *the child.* The ranks do not reflect the child's independence, as some mobility methods requiring less gross motor control (e.g., using a battery-powered wheelchair) may actually produce more independence than methods requiring more gross motor control (e.g., walking with an adult's hand). The ranks are not intended to imply that one mobility method is "better" or more efficient than another mobility method, but merely to reflect the motor control requirements of each method.

Using the construct of motor control, we calculated the actual ranks using data from the original population-based sample from the longitudinal study. Of the 682 children who had completed data at the first assessment (see subjects section), data from 354 children were used to calculate the ranks. These 354 children were classified at GMFCS Levels I-V and were ages 6-12 at the first assessment. Because the longitudinal study used a randomly selected population-based sample, the

TABLE 4. Ranks of Mobility Methods Used in the Home Setting

Rank	Mobility method used at home
1	Walks alone
2	Takes steps with walls/furniture
3	Walks with walking aid
4	Takes steps with adult hand
5	Rolls, creeps, crawls
6	Regular wheelchair
7	Battery-powered wheelchair
8	Carried by adult
9	Pushed by adult

sample was believed to be representative of the population of children with CP in Ontario, and potentially generalizable to populations elsewhere.

The ranks were based on the frequency (percentage) of mobility methods used in the home setting by children in each GMFCS level at the first assessment. The home setting was used as the basis for the ranking system because all nine mobility methods were used in the home. In addition, we believe that the home setting tends to have the least number of environmental obstacles, and may therefore provide a truer reflection of the child's motor control capability. The ranks were also calculated using the school and outdoors/community settings (data not shown) and the ranks were generally in the same order as the home setting.

For example, in order to calculate the rank for the mobility method, "battery-powered wheelchair," the following calculation was done: Data indicated that 19% of children in level IV and 1% of children in level V used a battery-powered wheelchair at home. No children in levels I - III used a battery-powered wheelchair at home. In order to weight the values according to GMFCS level (since GMFCS levels are intrinsically weighted in terms of gross motor function), the values were multiplied. For the mobility method "battery-powered wheelchair," the weighted value was 81 (calculated by multiplying 19 times 4, and 1 times 5, and totaling the sums). These weighted values were placed in order for all mobility methods, with the highest weighted value assigned the highest rank and the lowest value assigned the lowest rank.

By using values weighted by GMFCS level, the ranks reflect the gross motor function required by children to perform mobility methods. Mobility methods were therefore ranked higher (e.g., walking alone) when children in GMFCS levels I and II performed them. Mobility methods were ranked lower (e.g., pushed by an adult) when children in GMFCS levels IV and V performed them.

Changes in methods of mobility over time and across settings were analyzed using a two-way repeated measures ANOVA. Children from GMFCS levels II, II, and IV were analyzed together. The independent variables were time (with three levels: Times 1, 2, and 3) and setting (with three levels: home, school, and outdoors/community). The dependent variable was usual mobility method, converted into ranks. The sphericity assumption was tested using Mauchly's sphericity test (SPSS, 1999; Huck, 2000). For conditions where sphericity could not be assumed, the degrees of freedom were adjusted using the Huynh-Feldt correction (SPSS, 1999; Huck, 2000). Normality of the distribution of rank values was assessed for each time and setting using the skewness statistic provided by SPSS (SPSS, 1999). None of the nine skewness values was statistically significant, and none exceeded a fairly modest absolute value of 0.60. For significant effects, post hoc comparisons were conducted to determine the time intervals and settings that differed, using Bonferroni's corrections for multiple comparisons (Portney & Watkins, 2000).

RESULTS

Description of Mobility Methods

Table 5 describes the usual mobility methods across home, school, and community over the three time periods. The most commonly used mobility methods are presented. We defined commonly used methods as those used by four or more children in the sample, and therefore percentages do not always add to 100.

In the home setting, children most frequently used floor mobility or walked. At Time 1: 45% of children used rolling, creeping, or crawling, at Time 2: 37%, and at Time 3: 23%. At Time 1: 19% of children walked alone, at Time 2: 26%, and at Time 3: 23%. Other mobility methods reported in the home included walking with a walking aid and using a battery-powered wheelchair.

At school, children most frequently walked with a mobility aid or used power mobility. At Time 1: 34% of children used walking with a walking aid, at Time 2: 27%, and at Time 3: 23%. In addition, at Time 1: 21% of children used a battery-powered wheelchair, at Time 2: 24%, and at Time

TABLE 5. Usual Mobility Methods for Children in GMFCS Levels II-IV Across Time and Setting. The Percentages May Not Add to 100, as Only Those Mobility Methods Used by Four or More Children Are Reported.

	Time 1 (%) (N)	Time 2 (%) (N)	Time 3 (%) (N)
Home	Rolls, creeps, crawls 45% (28) Walks alone 19% (12) Walks with walking aid 11% (7) Battery-powered wheel-chair 8% (5)	Rolls, creeps, crawls 37% (23) Walks alone 26% (16) Walks with walking aid 11% (7) Battery-powered wheel-chair 8% (5)	Walks alone 26% (16) Rolls, creeps, crawls 23% (14) Walks with walking aid 18% (11) Battery-powered wheel-chair 11% (7)
School	Walks with walking aid 34% (21) Battery-powered wheel-chair 21% (13) Walks alone 15% (9) Regular wheelchair 15% (9) Pushed by an adult 15% (9)	Walks with walking aid 27% (17) Battery-powered wheel-chair 24% (15) Walks alone 23% (14) Regular wheelchair 16% (10) Pushed by an adult 7% (4)	Battery-powered wheel-chair 27% (17) Walks with walking aid 23% (14) Walks alone 21% (13) Regular wheelchair 13% (8) Pushed by adult 11% (7)
Outdoors/ community	Pushed by an adult 36% (22) Battery-powered wheel-chair 21% (13) Walks with walking aid 19% (12) Regular wheelchair 13% (8) Walks alone 10% (6)	Pushed by an adult 26% (16) Battery-powered wheel-chair 24% (15) Walks with walking aid 16% (10) Walks alone 16% (10) Regular wheelchair 13% (8)	Pushed by an adult 27% (17) Battery-powered wheel-chair 27% (17) Walks with walking aid 13% (8) Walks alone 13% (8) Takes steps with adult hand 10% (6) Regular wheelchair 8% (5)

3: 27%. Other usual mobility methods reported at school included walking alone, using a regular wheelchair, and being pushed by an adult.

In the outdoors/community, children most frequently used wheelchair mobility. At Time 1: 36% of children were pushed by an adult, at Time 2: 26%, and at Time 3: 27%. At Time 1: 21% of children used a battery-powered wheelchair, at Time 2: 24%, and at Time 3: 27%. Other usual mobility methods reported for the outdoors/community included walking with a walking aid, walking alone, using a regular wheelchair, and taking steps with an adult hand.

Overall Effect of Time and Setting on Mobility Methods

The two-way repeated measures ANOVA indicated a main effect for setting, $F(1.9, 116) = 39.3, p < 0.0001$ and a main effect for time,

F (1.7, 122) = 4.4, p = 0.02. The interaction of setting and time was not significant, F (3.4, 244) = .30, p = 0.86.

Post hoc comparisons for the *setting* main effect (data collapsed over time) indicated that there were significant differences between all three settings (Figure 2), based on the ranks of mobility methods from 1 (highest) to 9 (lowest). The unadjusted p-values are presented and using the Bonferroni correction would require a p < 0.0167 to be significant. In addition, 98.3% Confidence Intervals (CI) are presented to be consistent with a Bonferroni correction for the number of comparisons. At home, children used higher-ranked mobility methods (M = 4.01) than at school (M = 4.68): mean difference = .672 (98.3% CI = .217 to 1.127), SE = .185, t = 3.64, $p \le$ 0.001. At school, children used higher-ranked mobility methods (M = 4.68) than in the outdoors/community (M = 5.90): mean difference = 1.22 (98.3% CI = .679 to 1.762), SE = .220, t = 5.55, $p \le$ .0001. The mean difference between home (M = 4.01) and outdoors/community (M = 5.90) was significant: mean difference = 1.89 (98.3% CI = 1.30 to 2.485), SE = .241, t = 7.87, $p \le$ 0.0001. The comparison of the three settings, collapsed over time, was replicated with a Friedman rank ANOVA, followed by Bonferroni-corrected Wilcoxon

FIGURE 2. Estimated marginal means for mobility methods across time and settings. The top of the Y-axis represents higher-ranked mobility methods requiring more trunk and lower extremity motor control (e.g., walks with a walking aid is a rank of 3). The bottom of the Y-axis represents lower-ranked mobility methods requiring less motor control (e.g., uses a battery-powered wheelchair is a rank of 7).

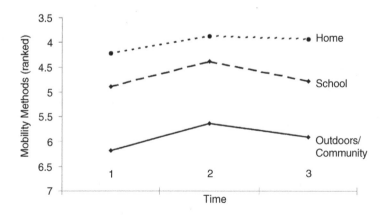

tests, due to the partially ordinal nature of the data. The results (overall $p \leq 0.0001$ and all three settings differed from each other at $p \leq 0.001$) were similar to the results from the parametric ANOVA.

There was a significant quadratic trend over time in the ANOVA (data collapsed across settings), $F(1, 61) = 12.2$, $p \leq 0.001$. This non-linear change over time is evident in Figure 2, as there was a different slope of change between the first time interval (Times 1 to 2) compared to the second time interval (Times 2 to 3). Post hoc contrasts for the time main effect indicated that there were significant differences in the first time interval: mean difference = .468 (98.3% CI = .110 to .825), $SE = .145$, $t = 3.22$, $p \leq 0.002$. At Time 2, children used higher-ranked mobility methods ($M = 4.63$) than at Time 1 ($M = 5.10$). The difference in the second time interval was not significant: mean difference = .242 (98.3% CI = .087 to .571), $SE = .134$, $t = 1.81$, $p = .075$, although both the significant non-linear time effect and the decreased marginal means indicate a trend towards lower-ranked mobility methods, especially in the school and outdoors/community. The difference between Time 1 and Time 3 was also not significant: mean difference = .226 (98.3% CI = .244 to .696), $SE = .191$, $t = 1.18$, $p = .242$. The comparison of the three time intervals, collapsed over setting, was replicated with a Friedman rank ANOVA followed by Bonferroni-corrected Wilcoxon tests, due to the partially ordinal nature of the data. Even though the overall Friedman ANOVA did not attain significance ($p = .145$), the results of the Wilcoxon tests were quite similar to the results from the t-tests used as follow-up to the parametric ANOVA. The Friedman test results may be an anomaly, as the data were fairly normally distributed and the Wilcoxon results parallel the parametric results. Furthermore, a non-parametric test does not account for a quadratic trend in the data, which was highly significant parametrically.

DISCUSSION

Children with CP, ages 6-14, classified at GMFCS levels II-IV demonstrated non-linear changes in usual mobility methods over a 3-4 year period. This study, being the first to examine longitudinal changes in mobility, provides some preliminary evidence of the changes in mobility methods over time. Usual mobility methods also differed across home, school, and outdoors/community settings, supporting previous research on the impact of the environment on mobility methods (Tieman, 2002; Palisano et al., 2003). These previous studies indicated that mobility methods used by children with CP vary across environmental settings. The interaction between time and setting (in the ANOVA) in this study was not statistically significant, suggesting that the pattern of change occurring in mobility over time may be similar across all settings. This issue should be examined in future studies with larger numbers of children and youth.

The results indicate that during the first time interval, mobility methods changed to mobility methods requiring more trunk and lower extremity control. There are a number of factors, both in terms of the child and the environment, that may influence these changes. These factors were not measured in this study, but should be explored further in future research. One possible explanation for the change in mobility methods in the first interval is the contribution of child-related changes in mobility. Child-related changes may include improved strength and endurance, motor learning (resulting from instruction and practice), or personal factors (such as motivation to keep up with peers). These factors may have enabled children to use mobility methods, such as walking alone or with a walking aid. During this first time interval there was, for example, an increase in the number of children walking alone. Perhaps these children became more proficient at walking alone, without mobility aids, and thus were able to utilize walking alone as their *usual* mobility method.

Environmental factors perhaps could have influenced the change to mobility methods requiring more motor control in the first time interval. The use of mobility methods requiring more motor control may suggest that environmental settings became more manageable over the first time interval. For example, the increase in the number of children walking alone may suggest that children became more adaptable in their environment and were able to use methods requiring more motor control. Another possible explanation of these findings is that modifications to improve physical accessibility and accommodations (including services and resources) may have facilitated use of mobility methods requiring more motor control (National Institutes of Health, 1993; Fougeyrollas, 1995; WHO, 2001). The details of the environmental factors were not examined in this study, but are important to study further in order to determine those factors contributing to changes in mobility.

During the second assessment interval, the results indicate a trend towards mobility methods requiring less trunk and lower extremity control, such as wheeled mobility. As with the first time interval, these changes are perhaps due to changes occurring within the child as well as within the environment. During this second time interval, for instance, there was a leveling off or decrease in the number of children walking alone. As children approach adolescence, the child-related changes impacting mobility may include increased body mass, secondary musculoskeletal impairments, and increased pain (Turk, 1994; Murphy, Molnar, & Lankasky, 1995). Several factors related to growth, such as weight gain, excessive forces through joints, and early joint degeneration, have been associated with decreased ability to walk during adolescence (Cathels & Reddihough, 1993; Turk, 1994; Murphy et al., 1995; Schwartz, Engel, & Jensen, 1999) and may have influenced use of mobility methods requiring less motor control. In addition to child-related changes, the environmental settings (especially school and outdoors/community) may have become more demanding (e.g., increased distances to classes, faster speeds, and increased social expectations), in comparison to the first time interval when children were younger and may have had less challenges in their elementary or middle school settings. In order to meet the increased demands of the environment, coupled with the child-related changes, children may have begun using mobility methods requiring less trunk and lower extremity motor control. For instance, the number of children using battery-powered wheelchairs increased during the second time interval. Perhaps children began using powered mobility because this mobility may be used continuously over time, despite changes that may occur within the child (e.g., musculoskeletal impairments) and within the environment (e.g., longer distances).

Many of the child and the environment factors that might contribute to changes in performance of mobility are associated with age. In this study, children ranged in age from 6 - 10 years at Time 1 and from 9 - 14 years at Time 3. The wide range of ages may have resulted in variability in the influence of growth and development, as children reach puberty at various ages. The children, ages 9 - 14 years at Time 3, may have been at various stages of growth changes related to puberty, as well as at different stages in middle or high school, which may have impacted mobility method. Future studies need to examine in more detail how physical growth and development influences performance of mobility of children with CP.

We had anticipated that the interaction (in the ANOVA) between time and setting would be significant, but in fact, the interaction was not statistically significant. We had expected to see greater changes in mobility over time in certain settings, such as school, outdoors, and community, and less changes in the home setting. The contextual features of each of these settings were not measured, so it is unknown how these features may have changed over time. For children who remained in the same home throughout the study, the contextual features (e.g., distances, time constraints, social expectations) of the home setting may not have changed as much as the school and outdoors/community settings. Over time, however, the school setting may have changed (e.g., from elementary to middle school) whereby it is assumed that the physical demands became greater with increased distances between classrooms, time demands in keeping up with peers, and increased social expectations. In addition, during late childhood and early adolescence, children often participate in recreational activities in more diverse outdoor and community settings such as sports fields, shopping malls, and movie theatres. Because of the increased environmental demands, both in the school and outdoors/community, children may have changed their mobility methods in order to keep up with peers. Future research should include measurement of contextual features of settings to explore whether changes in mobility occur more in certain settings.

Implications for Practice

The findings should assist physical therapists and occupational therapists in decision-making related to screening, examination, and intervention to improve mobility in children with CP. Screening is indicated during periods of transition within the child (e.g., rapid growth period) and within the environment (e.g., change of schools, new activities in the community), in order to determine if these changes affect mobility. If mobility has changed, an examination should be conducted to measure the changes within the child (e.g., capability, personal factors) and environment (e.g., features of the home, school, and outdoors/community). Depending on the results of examination, intervention may focus on the features of the child, the environment, or both. For example, physical and occupational therapy interventions may need to address musculoskeletal changes, fitness, architectural barriers, and technical accommodations in order to improve mobility. Interventions may be setting-specific depending on the person-environment interaction.

Previous research in the movement science literature (Gentile, 1987; Goodale, Jackobson, & Keillor, 1994) has emphasized the importance of learning and practicing a skill in the same setting where the skill will be used, since generalization may not occur across settings. The current study supports previous research (Tieman, 2002; Palisano et al., 2003) on the impact of environmental setting on usual mobility methods in children with CP. Children with CP, therefore, may need to learn and practice mobility methods specific to the environmental setting where they will use the skill. Further ecological studies are needed to explore the specific environmental features that may impact mobility, related to specificity of practice.

Physical and occupational therapy interventions may be indicated at specific points (i.e., episodes of care) throughout the lifespan of individuals with CP. Intervention should address age-related changes pertaining to growth and development and transitions to new environments. Physical and occupational therapy interventions should also include the prevention of secondary impairments (e.g., decreased endurance, joint degeneration) that may limit mobility in children as they become older (Campbell, 1997). In addition, new mobility equipment and training in the use of new equipment may be needed over time, and should be seen as facilitatory rather than as evidence of "failure."

CONCLUSION

The findings indicate that the mobility methods of children with CP change in a non-linear pattern over time and across settings. In the first assessment interval, mobility methods increased to mobility methods requiring more gross motor control. In the second assessment interval, mobility methods were unchanged or decreased to mobility methods requiring less gross motor control. These changes in mobility over time are hypothesized to be attributable to changes within the child (e.g., capability and personal factors), changes in the environment (e.g., contextual features) and changes in the person-environment interaction. We recommend that physical and occupational therapists should be attentive to the changes in the mobility of children with CP whenever changes occur within the child and/or the environment. Interventions to improve mobility in children with CP may need to occur at specific transition periods throughout the lifetime of an individual with CP. Future studies are needed to measure the specific factors, including the child factors and environmental features that contribute to the changes in mobility over time.

REFERENCES

Bax MCO. (1964). Terminology and classification of cerebral palsy. *Developmental Medicine and Child Neurology, 6,* 295-297.

Berry, E.T., McLaurin, S.E., & Sparling, J.W. (1996). Parent/caregiver perspectives on the use of power wheelchairs. *Pediatric Physical Therapy, 8,* 146-150.

Bottos, M., Dalla Barba, B., Stefani, D., Pettena, G., Tonin, C., & D'Este, A. (1989). Locomotor strategies preceding independent walking: Prospective study of neurological and language development in 424 cases. *Developmental Medicine and Child Neurology, 31,* 25-34.

Bottos, M., Puato, M.L., Vianello, A., & Facchin, P. (1995). Locomotion patterns in cerebral palsy syndromes. *Developmental Medicine and Child Neurology, 37*, 883-899.

Campbell, S.K. (1997). Therapy programs for children that last a lifetime. *Physical & Occupational Therapy in Pediatrics, 17*, 1-15.

Campos da Paz, A., Burnett S.M., & Braga, L.W. (1994). Walking prognosis in cerebral palsy: A 22-year retrospective analysis. *Developmental Medicine and Child Neurology, 36*, 130-134.

Cathels, B.A., & Reddihough, D.S. (1993). The health care of young adults with cerebral palsy. *Medical Journal of Australia, 159*, 444-446.

Fougeyrollas, P. (1995). Documenting environmental factors for preventing the handicap creation process: Quebec contributions relating to ICIDH and social participation of people with functional differences. *Disability and Rehabilitation, 17*(3-4), 145-153.

Gentile, A.M. (1987). Skill acquisition. Action, movement, and neuromotor processes. In: J.H. Carr and R.B. Shepher (Eds.), *Movement science: Foundations for physical therapy in rehabilitation.* (pp. 93-154). Rockville, MD: Aspen Publishers.

Glascoe, F.P. & Dworkin, P.H. (1995). The role of parents in the detection of developmental and behavioral problems. *Pediatrics, 95*(6), 829-836.

Goodale, M.A., Jackobson, L.S., & Keillor, J.M. (1994). Differences in the visual control of pantomimed and natural grasping movements. *Neuropsychologia, 32* (10), 1159-1178.

Haley, S.M., Coster, W.J., & Binda-Sundberg, K. (1994). Measuring physical disablement: The contextual challenge. *Physical Therapy, 74* (5), 443-451.

Huck, S.W. (2000). 3rd Ed. *Reading Statistics and Research,* New York: Addison Wesley Longman, Inc.

Law, M., Darrah, J., Pollock, N., King, G., Rosenbaum, P., Russell, D., Palisano, R., Harris, S., Armstrong, R., & Watt, J. (1998). Family-centered functional therapy for children with cerebral palsy: An emerging practice model. *Physical & Occupational Therapy in Pediatrics, 18 (1)*, 83-102.

Long, T.M. (1992). The use of parent report measures to assess infant development. *Pediatric Physical Therapy, 4*(2), 74-77.

Modell, S.J., Rider, R.A., & Menchetti, B.M. (1997). An exploration of the influence of educational placement on the community recreation and leisure patterns of children with developmental disabilities. *Perceptual and Motor Skills, 85*, 695-704.

Montgomery, P.C. (1998). Predicting potential for ambulation in children with cerebral palsy. *Pediatric Physical Therapy, 10*, 148-155.

Murphy, K.P., Molnar, G.E., & Lankasky, K. (1995). Cross-sectional description of the general health and of 101 adults aged between 19 and 74 years. *Developmental Medicine and Child Neurology, 37*, 1075-1084.

Mutch, L., Alberman, E., Hagberg, B., Kodama, K., & Perat, M.V. (1992). Cerebral palsy epidemiology: Where are we now and where are we going? *Developmental Medicine and Child Neurology, 34*(6), 547-51.

National Institutes of Health (1993). Research plan for the National Center for Medical Rehabilitation Research. NIH Publication No. 93-3509. Bethesda, MD: National Institutes of Health.

Palisano, R.J., Rosenbaum, P.L., Walter, S.D., Russell, D.J., Wood, E.P., & Galuppi, B.E. (1997). Development and reliability of a system to classify gross motor function in children with cerebral palsy. *Developmental Medicine and Child Neurology, 39,* 214-223.

Palisano, R.J., Hanna, S.E., Rosenbaum, P.L., Russell, D.J., Walter, S.D., Wood, E.P., Raina, P.S., & Galuppi, B.E. (2000). Validation of a model of gross motor function for children with cerebral palsy. *Physical Therapy, 80* (10), 974-985.

Palisano, R.J., Tieman, B.L., Walter, S.D., Bartlett, D.J., Rosenbaum, P.L., Russell, D., & Hanna, S.E. (2003). Effect of environment setting on mobility methods of children with cerebral palsy. *Developmental Medicine and Child Neurology, 45,* 113-120.

Pollock, N. & Stewart, D. (1990). A survey of activity patterns and vocational readiness of young adults with physical disabilities. *Canadian Journal of Rehabilitation, 4*(1), 17-26.

Pollock, N. & Stewart, D. (1998). Occupational performance needs of school-aged children with physical disabilities in the community. *Physical & Occupational Therapy in Pediatrics, 18,* 55-68.

Portney, L.G. & Watkins, M.P. (2000). 2nd ed. *Foundations of Clinical Research: Applications to Practice.* Norwalk, CT: Appleton and Lange.

Rosenbaum, P.L., Walter, S.D., Hanna, S.E., Palisano, R.J., Russell, D.J., Raina, P., Wood, E., Bartlett, D.J., & Galuppi, B.E. (2002). Prognosis for Gross Motor Function in Cerebral Palsy: Creation of Motor Development Curves. *Journal of the American Medical Association, 288*(11): 1357-1363.

Russell, D.J., Rosenbaum, P.L., Gowland, C., Hardy, S., Lane, M., Plews, N., McGavin, H., Cadman, D., & Jarvis, S. (1993). *Gross Motor Function Measure: A Measure of Gross Motor Function in Cerebral Palsy* (2nd ed.) Hamilton, Ontario: CanChild Centre for Childhood Disability Research.

Russell, D., Rosenbaum, P.L., Avery, L., & Lane, M. (2002). *The Gross Motor Function Measure (GMFM-66 and GMFM-88) User's Manual.* Clinics in Developmental Medicine, No. 159. London: MacKeith Press.

Schwartz, L., Engel, J.M., & Jensen, M.P. (1999). Pain in persons with cerebral palsy. *Archives of Physical Medicine and Rehabilitation, 80,* 1243-1246.

Scrutton, D. & Rosenbaum, P.L. (1997). The locomotor development of children with cerebral palsy. In K. Connolly & H. Forssberg (Eds.), *Neurophysiology and Neuropsychology Motor Development.* London: MacKeith Press.

Simeonsson, R.J., Lollar, D., Hollowell, J., & Adams, M. (2000). Revision of the International Classification of Impairments, Disabilities, and Handicaps: Developmental issues. *Journal of Clinical Epidemiology, 53,* 113-124.

SPSS 10.0.5 [Computer software]. (1999). Chicago, IL: SPSS Inc.

Tieman, B. (2002). *Usual mobility methods of children with cerebral palsy: A comparison across home, school, and outdoors/community settings.* Unpublished doctoral dissertation, MCP Hahnemann University (Drexel University), Philadelphia.

Trahan, J. & Marcoux, S. (1994). Factors associated with the inability of children with cerebral palsy to walk at six years: A retrospective study. *Developmental Medicine and Child Neurology, 36,* 787-795.

Turk, M.A. (1994). Attaining and retaining mobility: Clinical issues. In Lollar, D.J. (Ed.) *Preventing secondary conditions associated with spina bifida or cerebral* palsy. *Proceedings and Recommendations of a Symposium.* Washington, DC: Spina Bifida Association of America, 42-53.

Wilson, B.N., Kaplan, B.J., Crawford, S.G., Campbell, A., & Dewey, D. (2000). Reliability and validity of a parent questionnaire on childhood motor skills. *American Journal of Occupational Therapy, 54*(5), 484-493.

Wood, E. & Rosenbaum, P. (2000). The Gross Motor Function Classification System for cerebral palsy: A study of reliability and stability over time. *Developmental Medicine and Child Neurology, 42,* 292-296.

World Health Organization. (2001). *International Classification of Functioning, Disability, and Health (ICF)* Geneva: World Health Organization.

Young, N.L., Williams, J.I., Yoshida, K.K., Bombardier, C., & Wright, J.G. (1996). The context of measuring disability: Does it matter whether capability or performance is measured? *Journal of Clinical Epidemiology, 49,* 1097-1101.

Enhancing Prehension
in Infants and Children:
Fostering Neuromotor Strategies

Susan V. Duff
Jeanne Charles

SUMMARY. Learning to reach for and manipulate objects requires considerable neuromotor control and flexibility. Through environmental and object exploration individual neuromotor strategies expand, and prehensile skills improve, as infants and children overcome constraints.

Susan V. Duff, EdD, OTR/L, PT, CHT, BCP, is Research Associate, Clinical Research Department, Shriners Hospitals for Children, 3551 N. Broad Street, Philadelphia, PA 19140, and Clinical Faculty Associate, New York Medical College, School of Public Health, Program in Physical Therapy, Valhalla, NY USA (E-mail: sduff@shrinenet.org). Jeanne Charles, MSW, PT, is Project Manager, NIH- funded research project: The Effects of Constraint-Induced Therapy on Children with Cerebral Palsy, Movement Sciences Program, Department of Biobehavioral Sciences, Teachers College, Columbia University, 525 W. 120th Street, Box 199, New York, NY 10027 (E-mail: jrc44@columbia.edu).

The authors would like to extend their appreciation to Andrew M. Gordon, PhD, Professor, Movement Science Program, Department of Biobehavioral Sciences, Teachers College, Columbia University, for his keen advisement toward their doctoral degrees in Movement Science. They would also like to thank Gregory Murphy, MS, OTR/L, Ross Chavetz, MPH, PT, Megan Schaefer, DPT, and James C. Galloway, PT, PhD, for their thoughtful reviews of this article.

[Haworth co-indexing entry note]: "Enhancing Prehension in Infants and Children: Fostering Neuromotor Strategies." Duff, Susan V., and Jeanne Charles. Co-published simultaneously in *Physical & Occupational Therapy in Pediatrics* (The Haworth Press, Inc.) Vol. 24, No. 1/2, 2004, pp. 129-172; and: *Movement Sciences: Transfer of Knowledge into Pediatric Therapy Practice* (ed: Robert J. Palisano) The Haworth Press, Inc., 2004, pp. 129-172. Single or multiple copies of this article are available for a fee from The Haworth Document Delivery Service [1-800-HAWORTH, 9:00 a.m. - 5:00 p.m. (EST). E-mail address: docdelivery@haworthpress.com].

http://www.haworthpress.com/web/POTP
Digital Object Identifier: 10.1300/J006v24n01_06

Infants and children with prehensile deficits often have difficulty explor-
ing objects and the environment, thus, may not sufficiently develop the
strategies needed to expand their prehensile skills. This article reviews
neuromotor factors that influence prehension development, discusses
limitations to prehensile function and provides guidelines that can be
used to examine and enhance prehensile behaviors in infants and young
children based on a task-oriented approach addressing impairments, motor strategies and function. *[Article copies available for a fee from The
Haworth Document Delivery Service: 1-800-HAWORTH. E-mail address:
<docdelivery@haworthpress.com> Website: <http://www.HaworthPress.com>
© 2004 by The Haworth Press, Inc. All rights reserved.]*

KEYWORDS. Prehension, infancy, development, task-oriented approach, rehabilitation

Our limbs are the tools that enable us to make gestures, and engage in
age-specific purposeful activities. Prehension, or the use of the hands
and arms effectively, includes the components of visual regard, reach,
grasp, manipulation and release (see Duff, 2002 for review). The development of prehension can be challenging as infants learn to overcome
constraints within themselves and the environment (Thelen, 1998). Infants and children who are typically developing and those with congenital
or acquired disabilities meet this challenge by employing adaptive solutions. This article will: (1) review adaptability and other neuromotor
strategies that influence prehension development; (2) discuss problems
which limit prehensile function; and (3) suggest assessments and methods to evaluate and promote prehension in infants and children with motor delays or physical disabilities.

DEVELOPMENT OF PREHENSION

A neuromotor control perspective considers the biomechanical, neurological and environmental constraints which impact motor skills.
From this viewpoint the development of prehension involves an interaction between: (1) characteristics of the infant or child such as body
weight; (2) environmental features such as gravity; and (3) task goals
such as reaching for a hanging toy.

Prenatal and Infancy

Neuromotor factors that can influence prehension development include: adaptability, anticipatory control, unimanual/bimanual coordination, and object manipulation. Table 1 reviews how these overlapping factors impact prehension from the prenatal time period to early childhood.

Adaptability

Neural flexibility or adaptability is the ability to adjust, modify and transfer task performance based on limiting factors and changing conditions. The ability to adapt to intrinsic (internal) and extrinsic (external) constraints influences the development and expression of motor skills (Thelen, 1995). With experience, infants and children learn a range of solutions to different prehensile problems increasing their adaptive capacity. For example, to reach and grasp toys in different locations from varied body positions, they must learn to overcome gravity by engaging various muscle groups and movement patterns. The potential for prehensile skills developing with varied task and environmental demands should improve as adaptability increases.

Prenatal

Advances in technology have enabled researchers to examine characteristics of spontaneous fetal movements, as they transition into purposeful action behaviors (D'Elia et al., 2001; DiPetro et al., 2002; Kurjak et al., 2002; Robinson et al., 2000). For instance, ultrasound has been used to study upper limb *pre-natal* movement such as "thumb to mouth" activity in utero (deVries et al., 2001; McCartney & Hepper, 1999; Sparling et al., 1999). Sparling and colleagues (1997) suggest that fetal hand movements are not random and appear to be directed at targets. They also found that hand to face or hand to head movements at 32 weeks gestation were the best predictors of neonatal movement. Purposeful action behaviors may be the first signs of adaptability as the fetus begins to tailor his or her developing abilities to constraints in utero.

Infancy

Postnatal upper limb movements are considered to be random, yet evidence suggests that they are organized and can be adapted to various conditions. Amiel-Tison and Grenier (1980) stabilized the heads of ne-

TABLE 1. Neuromotor Strategies Influencing Prehension Development

	Prenatal	Early Infancy	Later Infancy	Early Childhood
Adaptability	• Purposeful action behaviors evident in utero may be first signs of adaptability	• Early movement strategies vary with differences in context, adaptability & physical traits. • Prehension development may not be restricted to an ontogenetic sequence	• Intrinsic and extrinsic factors along with experience influence the expression of prehension	• Ability to adjust to context & constraints expands with experience & development
Anticipatory Control	• Unknown	• Anticipatory visual tracking elicited • Anticipatory pre-shaping of the hand to object properties evident	• Improvement in anticipatory pre-shaping of the hand during reach • Anticipatory grading of grip force to conform to object properties emerges • Anticipatory postural adjustments (APA's) during reaching emerge	• Anticipatory control of hand pre-shaping & grading of fingertip forces continue to be refined • APA's prior to reaching continue to develop
Unimanual & Bimanual Coordination	• Pre-dominance of right or left unilateral movements are evident in utero	• Bimanual, symmetrical movement initially dominates • Early reaches are jerky & discontinuous • Gaze stabilization, head & trunk control precursors to skilled reaching • Feet reaching to objects precedes hand reaching	• Expression of unimanual & bimanual reaching varies due to interlimb coordination tendencies • Asymmetrical bimanual skill increasing	• Reaching path is smoother, more direct & adult-like • Refinement in symmetrical & asymmetrical bimanual skill continues
Object Manipulation	• Limited to own body due to confines of uterine environment • Grasp reflex develops	• Grasp reflex aids secure hold onto objects • Crude prehension patterns begin to form as infants begin to explore objects & the environment	• Repertoire of power & precision grasp patterns increase • As postural control & experience increase skilled manual function expands • Crude in-hand manipulation evident	• In-hand manipulation expands • Experience, interest, & attention dictate refinement

onates, providing postural support, and found the arm movements were less random and the infants seemed to reach toward objects. Hofsten and Ronnqvist (1993) quantified the random arm motion of young infants into movement units (one acceleration and one deceleration phase) and discovered that the arms seemed to move together or were temporally coupled. Kawai and colleagues (1999) examined the spontaneous arm movement of infants suspended in and out of water and in different positions (upright and supine). They found movements were more frequent out of the water and greater in the upright position. Thus, *context* such as postural support, body position and the environment plays an important role in the exhibition of early adaptive prehensile behavior.

As infants gain experience, matching behaviors to task demands and constraints, movement repertoires expand (see Table 1). Angulo-Kinzler and colleagues (2002) used the mobile paradigm introduced by Rovee-Collier and colleagues (Rovee-Collier & Sullivan, 1980; Sullivan et al., 1979) to document the adaptive kicking ability of 3-month-olds. They discovered that infants could move an overhead mobile by varying the kicking frequency or movement strategy employed, instead of relying on reciprocal kicking alone. Galloway and Thelen (in press) found lower limb reaching to precede upper limb reaching by about four weeks (which may reflect greater postural support). Thus, the legs and feet may potentially be employed as prehensile instruments, to explore objects sooner, than the arms and hands. In a study of "first" reaches in infants 12-22 weeks of age, Thelen and colleagues (1993) found infant reaching strategies to vary depending on individual physical traits and adaptive capacity. The ability to tailor limb movements to task demands and constraints early in life, suggests that young infants are not limited by hierarchical or sequential ontogenetic movement patterns.

Anticipatory Control

Neuromotor control of upper limb movement involves both feedback and anticipatory control. *Feedback* refers to sensory information gathered during movement. For example, during reaching, visual feedback ensures accurate finger opening and closure around objects at stable grasp points (Goodale et al., 1994; Jeannerod, 1990). However, feedback alone would be inefficient because we would have to wait for sensory input before adjusting to constraints. *Anticipatory control* involves advanced planning for task constraints or object properties and uses previous sensory information gained from experience to plan movement or prepare for postural perturbations (Hofsten, 1997; Johansson, 1996; Van der Fits et al., 1999b). For example, the first time we lift a heavy, slippery glass of water we may almost drop it since its weight and texture are unknown. But the second time, we usually can plan how much force to squeeze and lift with to prevent dropping it, because we are aware that it is heavy and slippery!

Anticipatory prehensile behavior has not been examined in the pre-natal period. However, postnatally, it has been shown during visual tracking and reach-to-grasp tasks (Hofsten & Fazel-Zandy, 1984; Hofsten & Lindhagen, 1979; Hofsten & Rosander, 1997; Rosander & Hofsten, 2000). By 5 months of age infants can *visually track* ahead of a moving target, predicting its future location (Hofsten & Rosander, 1997). Hofsten and Lindhagen (1979) found 18 week-old infants could intercept moving targets with the arms and hands displaying anticipatory *reach to grasp* behavior. By 13 months of age, infants demonstrate adult-like timing of grip formation (pre-shaping of the hand) to accommodate object properties (Hofsten & Ronnqvist, 1988).

Anticipatory control is also incorporated into postural adjustments and fingertip force scaling. Anticipatory postural adjustments (APA's) refer to stabilizing muscular contractions elicited in anticipation of expected disturbances in equilibrium. A high degree of postural activity, particularly in the neck region, is displayed by 4 to 5-month-old infants during goal-directed arm movements (Van der Fits et al., 1999a). Yet, it is not until 15 months of age that APA's are observed more consistently (Van der Fits et al., 1999b). Anticipatory control of fingertip forces used to grasp and lift objects begins to develop in late infancy and early childhood (Forssberg et al., 1992) as discussed in the section on *Object Manipulation*.

Unimanual/Bimanual Coordination

In the prenatal period the predominance of movement in one limb over the other may provide evidence for early *brain lateralization*. McCartney and Hepper (1999) found that from 12 to 27 weeks gestation, fetuses exhibited greater right-arm versus left-arm movements. The authors' postulated that this asymmetrical behavior directs later brain lateralization. Conversely, DeVries and colleagues (2001) studied the relationship between hand contact and head position in fetuses from 12 to 28 weeks gestation and did not find evidence of a lateralized preference.

In the neonatal period, bimanual upper limb movements predominate (Hofsten & Ronnqvist, 1993). While unimanual reaches are displayed, reaching is often bilateral (Rochat, 1992). Bimanual skill gradually improves as infants progress from midline play on the chest to hand to hand object transfer and bimanual voluntary reaching (Figure 1).

By four months of age, infants begin to reach and grasp objects (Spencer & Thelen 2000; Van der Fits et al., 1999a). These early reaches are variable, jerky movements (Konczak & Dichgans, 1997; Thelen, 1998; Thelen et al., 1996). Yet, as infants learn to overcome constraints and increase practice time, reaching becomes smoother and more consis-

FIGURE 1. Four-month-old displaying bimanual reach to grasp behavior toward a hanging toy.

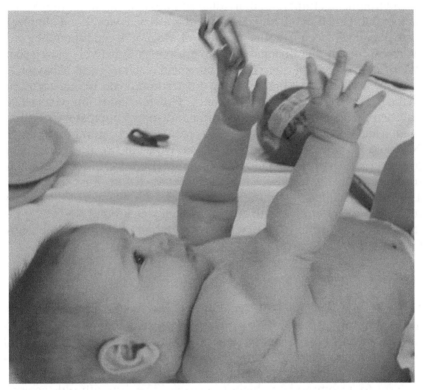

Printed with permission.

tent (Thelen, 1998). Konczak and Dichgans (1997) examined reaching in infants 5 months to 3 years of age and found that initially reaches were segmented, with a display of multiple velocity peaks. By 2 years of age, reaching was smoother with children displaying single velocity peaks.

Important precursors to successful reaching are gaze stabilization, head and trunk postural control and coordination (Bertenthal & Hofsten, 1998; Thelen & Spencer, 1998; Van der Fits & Hadders-Algra, 1998). Improvements in postural control and coordination enhance the accuracy and efficiency of reaching in various body positions (Corbetta & Thelen, 1996; Fallang et al., 2000; Van der Fits & Hadders-Algra, 1998). Corbetta and colleagues (Corbetta & Bojczyk, 2002; Corbetta & Thelen, 1996) postulated that in the first year, infants fluctuate between unimanual and bimanual reaches due to changes in interlimb coordination tendencies and balance demands, as exemplified during early walking.

Environmental limits and individual abilities also influence the expression of unimanual or bimanual reach and grasp behavior. For example, if a small ball is placed near the shoulder of a 7-month-old infant they will typically employ a unimanual reach to grasp it. Alternatively, a large ball placed in midline will often elicit a bimanual reach to grasp behavior.

Grip formation during reaching to accommodate object size and shape begins to develop during infancy. Hofsten and Ronnqvist (1988) reported that 5-month-old infants did not display anticipatory grip formation and opened their hand wide to receive objects, minimizing error. Nine and 13-month-old infants, however, were able to adjust their hand to object size before contact. The timing between grip formation and reaching gradually improves into adolescence (Kuhtz-Buschbeck et al., 1998a-b). In adults, the timing of peak hand opening (aperture) during a reach is loosely coupled with the reach, occurring around 70-75% of the total movement time from reach onset to target contact (Jackobson & Goodale, 1991; Jeannerod, 1984).

Object Manipulation

Grasp reflexes and simple hand movements enable the fetus to initiate exploratory gestures. Postnatally, early visual and manual exploration of objects helps the infant gain information about specific physical properties such as shape, size, texture and weight. Newell and colleagues (1989) found that 4 and 8-month-old infants could adapt grip patterns to accommodate object properties. The 4-month-olds seemed to obtain object information through *haptic (stereognosis)* and *visual exploration* while the 8-month-olds relied primarily on vision. Bimanual coordination initially is symmetrical then progresses to asymmetrical skill as the hands begin to employ different roles. By 12-18 months of age, one hand can actively stabilize while the other hand manipulates an object.

Power and *precision grip* patterns expand with neural development and the opportunity for exploration and practice. Power grips transmit forces from the fingers and thumb against the palm and precision grips transmit forces between the fingers and thumb (Napier, 1956). As experience widens and the connection between the motor neuronal pool and cortex is strengthened, isolated finger movement and precision grip patterns such as the pincer grasp develop (Hirschel et al., 1990; Forssberg et al., 1991).

Adult-like object manipulation incorporates *anticipatory control* and *sensory feedback* (Johansson & Cole, 1992). *Internal representations* of object properties are formed from past experience and retrieved from *memory* to grade fingertip forces in advance of contact (anticipatory control). Internal representations are used to plan *grip (squeeze)* and *load (lift) forces* in advance of contact, to prevent damage from gripping too tightly or lifting too quickly (Gordon et al., 1993; Johansson & Westling, 1984, 1987, 1988; Westling & Johansson, 1987). Sensory feedback during lifts provides information about object contact and weight and is used to upgrade the grip or load force if the object slips. Following lifts, tactile and proprioceptive feedback is used to update memory systems to object texture and weight. Young infants cannot adequately control fingertip forces and may crush fragile objects such as a paper cup or fail to lift heavy ones such as a ceramic cup. By 18 months to two years of age, anticipatory control during object manipulation begins to develop (Forssberg et al., 1992).

Early Childhood

During early childhood, neuromotor strategies are refined as children gain strength and engage in peer-related play activities and task specific practice. While the path of upper limb reaching becomes smoother and more direct by two years of age (Konczak & Dichgans, 1997), anticipatory grip formation does not become adult-like until adolescence (Kuhtz-Buschbeck et al., 1998a-b). Postural adjustments employed in anticipation of going off balance during reaching tasks in standing are well developed by 4-6 years of age (Woollacott & Shumway-Cook, 1986). Bimanual coordination continues to expand as the child gains experience with symmetrical (e.g., ball throwing) or asymmetrical tasks (e.g., cutting with scissors while holding paper). During this period object manipulation skills expand considerably.

During object manipulation, the two-year-old child displays some anticipatory control of fingertip forces during object lifts, yet they continue to rely on tactile and proprioceptive feedback to enhance success (Forssberg et al., 1992, 1995). Specifically, they may push down on objects before lifting them or demonstrate multiple attempts to lift before successfully raising an object off its support surface. However, by 6-8 years of age, force scaling, using both anticipatory and feedback control, approaches that of adults (Forssberg et al., 1992, 1995).

As prehension patterns and pencil grips form (Erhardt, 1971; Schneck & Henderson, 1990) and fingertip force scaling becomes more refined, *in-hand manipulation*, or the ability to move objects in one hand, is developed. Elements of in-hand manipulation include: (1) *translation* or moving objects between the palm and fingers; (2) *shift* or adjusting the position of a held object by the fingertips; and (3) *rotation* or turning an object on its center axis (Exner, 1990). Crude in-hand manipulation may develop early, given evidence that 8-month-old infants can hold a rod with the ulnar digits and manipulate it with the radial thumb and index fingers (Lantz et al., 1996). However, competence, as found during complex rotation (180 degrees), is not seen until 3-4 years of age (Exner, 1993). With practice, a child can quickly bring a pencil from the palm to the fingertips, move the fingers toward the tip or rotate it to use the eraser.

Practice influences the acquisition of motor skills (Gentile, 1998; Lobo et al., submitted, per conversation). Initially, the shape/structure or general form of a movement is performed, and after sufficient practice, the components and timing are refined, leading to the attainment of the skill (Gentile, 1998). Prehensile behaviors displayed by those with disabilities will differ from those of typically developing children, yet if adaptability and other neuromotor strategies can be fostered during practice, function may be enhanced (Charles et al., 2001).

PROBLEM IDENTIFICATION

Unconventional or compensatory methods to accomplish functional tasks may not be as efficient yet they often enhance success. Given this, how do therapists decide when to intervene? Furthermore, how are the prognosis and projected outcomes from intervention for a particular infant or child determined? In their chapter on evidenced-based practice, Depoy and Gitlow (2001) suggest the following sequence be used as a guide to evaluation and intervention:

1. Identify the *problem*: Determine cause and consequences;
2. Determine the *need* (s): With evidence obtained through assessment;
3. Set *goals* and objectives;
4. Implement *intervention*; and
5. Establish the process and *outcome* assessment.

Regardless of the scenario, the child, family and therapist must determine and prioritize the problem(s) and need(s) based on a thorough assessment. After priorities are established, the therapist and family can decide whether intervention is warranted. The goals and objectives are then determined and will direct the type of intervention and outcome measures used. In this section potential problems in adaptability, anticipatory control, unimanual and bimanual coordination, and object manipulation are discussed.

Limited Adaptability

Thelen (1995) proposed that neuromotor behaviors displayed by children with neurological deficits reflect their capacity to adapt to inherent environmental and tasks constraints. Infants and children with congenital or acquired differences may have a small repertoire of prehensile strategies available. While a limited repertoire may be sufficient if task components or the environment do not change, performance may be impacted if there are alterations to the task or context. For example, a 2-year-old with arthrogyposis may be able to bring a fork to her mouth to eat by sliding the arm across a chest-high table using shoulder musculature. This action would subsequently passively flex the elbow through intersegmental processes, bringing the hand to the mouth. However, if the fork is changed to a spoon and the table height is lowered, the child may be unsuccessful at acquiring and retaining the food since he/she cannot actively supinate the forearm or flex the elbow.

Impaired Anticipatory Control

Anticipatory control, used to maintain balance, preshape the hand or grade fingertip forces to accommodate object properties, is refined with experience. Children with unilateral deficits such as hemiplegic cerebral palsy and Erb's palsy have limited experience manipulating objects with their involved hand, and children with arthrogryposis often have bimanual limitations (Hahn, 1985). This limited experience may impact the development of anticipatory control.

Impaired sensory feedback may also impact anticipatory control leading to compensatory behaviors such as delayed postural responses or inefficient grasp and manipulation as found in children with hemiplegic cerebral palsy (Gordon & Duff, 1999a-b; Hadders-Algra et al., 1999). Hadders-Algra and colleagues (1999) found that while the basic organization of postural adjustments was intact in children with cerebral palsy, they could not adapt them to task specific constraints. Children with hemiplegic cerebral palsy exhibit time delays during reach to grasp tasks (Eliasson et al., 1991; Steenbergen et al., 1998). These children often exaggerate grip formation by hyperextending the metacarpophalangeal joints in the involved hand and prolonging the time taken to make accurate finger contact on objects. Also, during object manipulations, the rate of force is not adjusted to the object's properties. Children with hemiplegic cerebral palsy often employ excessive grip or squeeze force and negative instead of positive load forces (Eliasson et al., 1992, 1995). While compensatory behaviors can lead to successful attainment of task goals, they often result in inefficient prehensile strategies.

Restricted Unimanual and Bimanual Coordination

Physical impairments such as reduced strength, limited range-of-motion, pain, or high/low muscle tone can limit unimanual and bimanual exploration of objects and the environment. For instance, infants with unilateral conditions such as Erb's palsy may avoid turning the head to the affected side, leading to neck contractures, further limiting visual exploration and arm movement on that side (Ramos & Zell, 2000). Infants with arthrogryposis have joint contractures and restricted muscle activation that can limit reaching and other gross motor skills (Hahn, 1985; Palmer et al., 1985).

Unilateral weakness and joint contractures found in children with neurological or orthopedic deficits (Gordon & Duff, 1999a-b; Ramos & Zell, 2000; Waters, 1997) might restrict performance in age appropriate tasks such as prone propping in infancy, activities of daily living (ADL) and sports. These children often display atypical reaching patterns (Figure 2) or avoid using the involved limb, relying on the non-involved limb for most tasks. While reaching in the involved arm of children with hemiplegic cerebral palsy is reportedly enhanced during bimanual tasks (Utley & Sugden, 1998), slowness and control issues may hinder overall coordination.

Restricted Object Manipulation

Although impaired anticipatory control, timing and release do not prevent children from grasping and manipulating objects, the compensatory behaviors used to perform tasks may reduce movement efficiency and smoothness. Without accurate internal representations of objects, children tend to rely on these behaviors and thus may drop slippery objects or crush fragile ones. Children with hemiplegic cerebral palsy have documented impairments in sensibility in both hands

FIGURE 2. An atypical unimanual reaching pattern elicited in this 4-month-old with Erb's palsy with limited active shoulder external rotation and strong internal rotation.

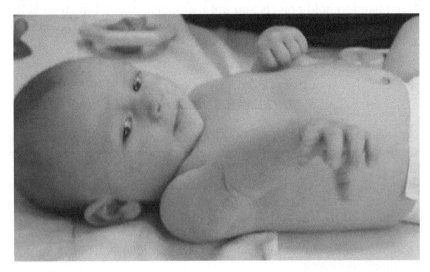

Printed with permission.

(Eliasson et al., 1992; Gordon & Duff, 1999b) that are associated with limitations in object manipulation including grading of fingertip forces as reviewed earlier (Gordon & Duff, 1999b).

Object manipulation is also limited by incomplete finger isolation needed for precision grip, in-hand manipulation and release of objects (Brown, 1967; Gordon et al., 2003; Hahn, 1985). Incomplete finger isolation and in-hand manipulation may stem from poorly developed corticomotoneuronal connections (Bennett & Lemon, 1996; Kuypers, 1978), strength deficits (Brown, 1967) or contractures as found in children with arthrogryposis (Hahn, 1985). Gordon and colleagues (Eliasson & Gordon, 2000; Gordon et al., 2003) examined release in children with hemiplegic cerebral palsy and found that they often release objects abruptly onto support surfaces and prolong the reduction in fingertip forces and finger release. To compensate, these children often use the non-involved hand to remove objects from the involved hand or rely on the *tenodesis* effect (fingers extend when the wrist flexes) (Erhardt, 1982).

Children with Erb's palsy usually have minimal limitations in hand function (Waters, 1997). However, unimanual or bimanual performance may be uncoordinated or inefficient if active supination, elbow flexion or shoulder motion is restricted in the involved limb. Because children with Erb's palsy or hemiplegic cerebral palsy often use the involved hand to hold objects and not manipulate them, bimanual skills may be confined to tasks that require the non-involved hand to serve as the manipulator and the involved hand to act as a stabilizer.

ASSESSMENT AND EVALUATION: DETERMINING NEED

A *task-oriented approach* to clinical care was created by Shumway-Cook and Woollacott (2001) based on review of various models of disablement (Nagi, 1965; NCMRR, 1992; WHO, 1980). This approach can be used to examine and treat prehensile deficits within a given disabling condition from three levels: (1) function; (2) motor strategy; and (3) impairment (Duff et al., 2001). The components of the approach are defined as:

- *Impairment*: neuromuscular or musculoskeletal constraints to functional movement.
- *Motor Strategy*: neuromotor control used to achieve functional tasks or activities.
- *Function*: the ability to perform essential tasks and activities.

Table 2 (A-C) reviews the problems often identified with Erb's palsy, arthrogryposis multiplex congenita (arthrogryposis), and hemiplegic cerebral palsy from a task-oriented approach.

While numerous assessments exist, some are better suited to assess the prehension of young infants and children with a range of disabling conditions. Examples of tools at each level of the task-oriented approach are listed in Tables 3 to 5. The measures listed in the tables are not inclusive. Rather they represent measures that we have found useful in our practice and research. Sample assessments suitable for use in children with Erb's palsy, arthrogryposis, or hemiplegic cerebral palsy are listed in Table 6.

Function

Functional evaluations measure the ability to perform everyday activities. Table 3 lists sample tests that can be used to assess upper limb and hand function in infants and children. The Jebsen-Taylor Test of Hand Function (Jebsen et al., 1969; Taylor et al., 1973) is one of the

TABLE 2. Task-Oriented Approach to Problem Identification

A: *Erb's Palsy*

Impairments	Motor Strategy Limits	Functional Limitation
• Proximal muscle weakness • Restricted repertoire of movement in involved upper limb	*Adaptability* • Limited unilateral reaching strategies • Inefficient bimanual movements	• Play (environmental & object exploration) • Bimanual tasks
• Visual neglect, painful neck rotation • Possible sensibility deficits	*Anticipatory Control* • Potential limitation	• May have difficulty locating objects
• Absent or weak shoulder ER elevation & elbow flexion • Secondary joint contractures	*Unimanual & Bimanual Coordination* • Limited reaching strategies • Restricted bimanual strategies	• Difficulty with ADL tasks using involved hand • Bimanual task function restricted
• Slightly weak grip strength, forearm supination, elbow flexion • Forearm-elbow contractures	*Object Manipulation* • Limited skilled bimanual function • Inefficient compensatory strategies	• Greater impact on bimanual manipulation if forearm supination is lacking

B: *Arthrogryposis*

Impairments	Motor Strategy Limits	Functional Limitation
• Limited muscle activation • Joint contractures • Restricted movement repertoire	*Adaptability* • Limited prehensile strategies • Limited problem-solving experiences	• Dependent in many ADL tasks • Significant limits for play
• Limited neck mobility • Potential sensibility deficits • Potential deficit in internal representation of objects • Slow, labored movements • Weakness, joint contractures	*Anticipatory Control* • Minimal impact • Inability to pre-shape hand during reach • Impaired grading of fingertip forces during grasp & release	• Infants may have difficulty exploring & locating objects • Neck mobility & weakness limit unimanual/ bimanual play & ADL
• Slow, labored movements • Weakness, joint contractures	*Unimanual & Bimanual Coordination* • Limited reach to grasp strategies • Inefficient compensatory strategies	• Limits for play & ADL
• Weak grip/joint contractures • Limited prehension patterns • Diminished sensibility	*Object Manipulation* • May be unable to grasp smaller objects • Limited or absent in-hand manipulation	• Extreme difficulty with object manipulation for play & ADL

earliest assessments of upper limb function. Other tools such as the Pediatric Evaluation of Disability Inventory (PEDI) (Haley et al., 1992), School Function Assessment (SFA) (Coster et al., 1998) and the Wee-FIM (Msall et al., 1994) measure "what the child *does*" in his/her environment versus "what they *can do*" and thus provide a measure of *participation*. Select tools, such as handwriting assessments (Benbow, 1995; Amundson, 1995), are used to target specific problem areas.

TABLE 2 (continued)

C. *Hemiplegic Cerebral Palsy*

Impairments	Motor Strategy Limits	Functional Limitations
• Weakness, spasticity, incoordination in the involved limb promote disuse • Limited movement repertoire	**Adaptability** • Limited & less efficient unilateral & bimanual prehensile strategies	• Limited (environmental & object exploration) • Limited bimanual tasks
• Possible visual neglect / perceptual deficits • Diminished sensibility • Distorted internal representations of object properties	**Anticipatory Control** • Inaccurate hand pre-shaping & APA's • Impaired grading of fingertip forces during grasp & release	• Difficulty locating objects • Visual-perceptual deficits limit function • Reduced ADL efficiency
• Weak involved limb, spasticity, secondary joint contractures • Slower/uncoordinated movements	**Unimanual & Bimanual Coordination** • Repertoire of reaching & bimanual strategies reduced or inefficient	• Unimanual & bimanual ADL & play tasks with involved limb are difficult
• Weak grip strength • Limited prehension patterns • Impaired pre-shaping of hand & grading of grip force • Excess tone finger/wrist flexors • Diminished sensibility	**Object Manipulation** • Difficulty with large or heavy objects • May be unable to open hand wide enough to grasp objects or unable to "let go" once held • Limited or absent in-hand manipulation	• Difficulty with object manipulation during ADL performance • Bimanual manipulative tasks difficult or inefficient

Along with determining functional ability, many tools also provide the opportunity to examine problem solving, movement efficiency and the range of prehension patterns available.

Some scales designed for use with adults or older children can be modified for infants. For instance, the Motor Activity Log (MAL) (Taub & Wolf, 1997) is a non-standardized scale used to monitor improvement in motor activity in adults recovering from stroke and in children with hemiplegic cerebral palsy following "constraint-induced movement therapy" (CIT) (Charles et al., 2001; Taub, 1993). It is sensitive to change (Charles et al., 1999; Page et al., 2001; Sterr et al., 2002) and could be adapted for use with older infants who display unimanual disuse, using such tasks as holding a bottle, securing finger food from a tray or pulling oneself to stand.

While functional assessments are useful to document ability, they do not always provide the insight behind the difficulty. Evaluation of motor strategies (e.g., anticipatory control) and impairments (e.g., weakness) may provide that additional information.

TABLE 3. Tools to Measure Prehensile Function

Tool	Description	Measurement Criteria	Age Range	Reference(s)
Developmental Skill Observations of the "K" & "1" Child Observations for Cursive Handwriting Skills Training	Functional handwriting assessment	Legibility, speed, pencil management & copying	Children in Kindergarten & First grade	Benbow, 1995
Evaluation Tool of Children's Handwriting (ETCH)	Functional handwriting assessment	Legibility, speed, pencil management & copying	School-age	Amundson, 1995
Jebson-Taylor Test of Hand Function	Designed to simulate hand function common to many ADL tasks	Timed subtests	Standardized 4-21 years	Jebsen et al., 1969, Taylor et al., 1973.
Motor Activity Log for Children	Caregiver survey of age appropriate, bimanual & unimanual usage	5-point Likert scale 1) Amount of Use 2) Quality of Movement	Non-standardized	Charles et al., 1997 Taub, 1993
Pediatric Evaluation of Disability Inventory (PEDI)	Standardized Test of Function/Clinician Examination and Caregiver Assessment (measures participation)	• Criterion referenced scale • Direct observation and/or interview of a parent or caregiver	6 months to 7.5 years	Haley et al., 1992
School Function Assessment (SFA)	Standardized Test designed to identify strengths and limitations in school related functional tasks in participation, task supports & activity performance	• Scale 1-4 • Direct observation and/or interview of a teacher or school-based therapist	Kindergarten to 6th grade	Coster et al., 1998
Wee-FIM System® Version 5.1 Motor Activity Log for Children	Determines child's consistent & usual performance to criterion standards of essential self-care, bowel & bladder management, locomotion, transfers, communication & social cognition	• 7-level Criterion referenced ordinal scale • Direct observation and/or interview of a parent or caregiver	• Non-disabled children: 6 months to 7 years • Disabled children: 6 months to 21 years	Guide for the Functional Independence Measure for Children 1993; Msall et al., 1994

Motor Strategies

This level of the evaluation examines neuromotor strategies inherent in prehension including: adaptability, anticipatory control, unimanual/bimanual coordination and object manipulation. The method of assessment for these components typically includes observation, video-recording or timing using videocoding or a stopwatch. Since few assessments are specifically designed to measure motor strategies, a review of non-standardized methods has also been provided.

TABLE 4. Tools to Measure Prehensile Motor Strategies

Tool	Description	Measurement Criteria	Age-Range	References
Bayley Scales of Infant Development®, 2nd Ed (BSID-II)	Fine-motor section of Motor Scale	Ordinal scale	1-42 months	Bayley, 1993
Bruininks-Oseretsky Test of Motor Proficiency: Fine Motor Subtest	Evaluates upper limb coordination, response speed, visual-motor control, & dexterity	Criterion referenced descriptive scale	4.5 -16.5 years	Bruinicks, 1978
Erhardt Developmental Prehension Assessment	Grasp pattern assessment	Criterion referenced descriptive scale	Birth to 6 years	Erhardt, 1982
Fingertip Force Scaling	Measures gradation of grip & lift forces during object manipulation	Descriptive unless kinetic fingertip force measures are recorded	Non-specific	Forssberg et al., 1991, 1992, 1995; Eliasson et al., 1991, 1992, 1995; Gordon & Duff, 1999a-b; Gordon et al., 1999, 2003
Gaze Stabilization & Following	Observe or videotape visual attention, saccadic eye movements, pursuit, bilateral eye function & gaze stability during head & trunk movement	Grade as intact, impaired or unable	Non-specific	Herdman et al., 2001; Galloway et al., 2002
In-Hand Manipulation	Measures translation, shift, & rotation of objects in one-hand	Descriptive	Standardization incomplete	Exner, 1990; Pehoski, 1995
Miller Assessment for Preschoolers™ (MAP™)	Measures sensori-motor abilities in conjunction with cognitive abilities	Descriptive	2.9 to 5.8 years	Miller, 1988
Reaching to Stationary or Moving Target	Observe or videotape reach to grasp of targets then analyze timing of select segments	• Descriptive • Timed measures • Kinematic analysis	Non-specific	Jeannerod, 1981
Peabody Fine Motor Scale	Evaluates reflexes, hand-use, eye-hand coordination, & manual dexterity	Ordinal scale	Birth to 7 years	Folio & Fewell,1983; Cohen et al., 1999
Quality of Upper Extremity Skills Test (QUEST)	Evaluates quality in 4 domains: dissociated movement, grasp, protective extension, & weight bearing	Criterion referenced scale	18 months to 8 years	DeMatteo et al., 1993
Sollerman's Grip Test	Evaluation of select prehension patterns	4-point ordinal scale	Non-specific	Sollerman, 1984

TABLE 5. Tests to Measure Prehensile Impairment

Tool	Description	Measurement Criteria	Age-Range	References
Active Movement Scale (AMS)	Tests active unimanual movement of infants in gravity-eliminated & against gravity positions	8-point ordinal scale	Non-standardized yet designed to test infants with brachial plexus birth palsy	Clarke & Curtis, 1995; Curtis et al., 2002
Beery-Buktenica Test of Visual-Motor Integration	Tests visual-motor ability to copy 3-D designs and integration of perceptual cues	3-point scoring criteria for each figure drawn	2-15 years yet primarily designed for children in preschool & early elementary school	Beery, 1997
Dynamometer and Pinchmeter	Isometric grip & pinch strength	Kilograms or pounds	Non-specific	Mathowitz et al., 1986; Fess, 1992
Manual Form Perception Test (from SIPT)	Evaluates stereognosis via matching of various plastic shapes held in the hand against a picture card with vision occluded from view of the shape	Matching shapes felt in hand to 2-D paper design	Standardized on children 4-8 years	Sensory Integration & Praxis Test (Ayres, 1989)
Manual Muscle Test	Grading of muscle strength with isometric or isotonic tests	5 grades	Non-specific	Clarkson & Gilewich, 2000
Moberg Picking-Up Test	Manual placement of objects with or without vision occluded	Timed test	Non-specific	Dellon, 1981
Modified Ashworth Scale	Tests passive response to stretch as measure of spasticity	0-4 ordinal scale	Non-specific	Bohannon & Smith, 1987
Motor Free Visual Perceptual Test-Revised	2-D non-motor test of visual discrimination, visual form constancy, gestalt perception, visual matching, & visual memory	Matching of test designs	Standardized, 4-11 years	Colarusso & Hammill, 1996
Range-of-Motion (ROM)	Angle measurement of active & passive range-of-motion available at joints	Angle in degrees using goniometer	Non-specific	Clarkson and Gilewich, 2000
Semmes Weinstein Monofilament Test	Evaluates pressure sensitivity	Log_{10} grams of force	Non-specific	Weinstein, 1993; Stone, 1992
Test of Visual-Perceptual Skills (TVPS-R)	2-dimensional test of visual perception	Matching of test designs	Standardized, 4-12 years	Gardner, 1996
Two-Point Discrimination	Evaluates the ability to discriminate between one & two points	Distance between two points in mm	Non-specific	Stone, 1992

TABLE 6. Sample Assessments for Three Conditions Using a Task-Oriented Approach

	Function	Motor Strategies	Impairments
3-month-old with Erb's palsy	• Play & exploratory behaviors • Tolerance to various positions	• Gaze fixation & following • Observation or video-recording of arm flapping, early reaching to objects	• Active Movement Scale • Passive Range-of-Motion (PROM) • Arm posture at rest
2-year-old with Arthrogryposis	• Play & exploratory behaviors • WEE-FIM System® Version 5. • Pediatric Evaluation of Disability Inventory (PEDI) • Screen ability to use switch toys	• Bayley Scale • Observation or video-recording of reaching, object manipulation toward objects • Alter prehensile demands by changing positions	• Modified Active Movement Scale instead of manual muscle test • Active & PROM • Posture of arms at rest • Gross sensibility measure using an eraser
7-year-old with hemiplegic CP	• Motor Activity Log • School Function Assessment (SFA) • Jebsen-Taylor Test of Hand Function • Pediatric Evaluation of Disability Inventory (PEDI)	• Observation or video-recording of reach to grasp, object manipulation with & without wrist support • Sollerman's grip test • Bruinicks-Oseretsky Test	• Manual muscle test • Grip & pinch strength • Active & PROM • Sensibility tests • Arm posture at rest • Screen vision & visual-perception skills

Adaptability

There are no standardized tests of adaptability. The best way to gain insight into adaptability is to alter task components or introduce a new context. For example, an infant with Erb's palsy lying in supine could be presented with a toy on the involved side of the body directly in front of the chest. If they successfully grasp the toy, the therapist could change the size and type of toy (to demand a change in grip formation and grip pattern), the location (to demand they reach in a different plane) or change the position of the infant (from supine to semi-supported). Adaptability can be inferred by specifying the object's location, body position and response time.

Anticipatory Control

Although kinematic (spatial-temporal) analysis may be the ideal way to examine anticipatory behavior, observation and videotaped time-coding may be the most cost-effective and efficient methods available. Anticipatory postural adjustments include muscle contractions elicited to prevent one from going off balance. They can be assessed by engaging a child in activities that require timed ball throwing and catching. Anticipatory reaching behavior includes the ability to reach toward the future location of an object and correctly pre-shape the hand to accommodate object properties. Problems that can be revealed through assessment of anticipatory postural adjustments or reaching include inefficient timing of movement components, lost equilibrium, and inaccurate hand opening or closure on an object. For these tasks, mats ensure safety and balls and objects of various sizes, shapes and texture help gauge ability.

Anticipatory fingertip force scaling involves grading of forces in advance of object contact. Ideally, multi-axial force transducers are used to assess force scaling. However, because, the technique is cost-prohibitive, videotaped observation may be the only method available. A range of objects from light to heavy and fragile to stable (e.g., styrofoam vs. hard plastic) could be used to test ability. Problems that may be revealed through assessment include object slippage or excessive squeezing (grip force). Also, if the rate of load force onset is inefficient, the object(s) may be lifted too fast or too slow.

Unimanual and Bimanual Coordination

Spontaneous arm movements (flapping) and reach to grasp behaviors can be analyzed by counting the frequency of occurrence (Galloway et al., 2002) or by using kinematics (Lobo et al., submitted). Unimanual or bimanual reach to grasp in older infants and children can be analyzed by recording the total movement time or a subcomponent using a stopwatch (or time code on videotape) (Jeannerod, 1981). When evaluating reach to grasp ability, it is important to document whether the target object is stationary or moving, and to note its size and contour. Problems that might be revealed through examination include prolonged time to reach the object, an awkward hand path exhibited toward the object, or poor arm coupling during symmetrical bimanual tasks.

In addition to behavioral observations, bimanual coordination can be examined using timed measures as found in the Fine-Motor Subtest of the Bruininks-Oseretsky Test of Motor Proficiency (Bruinicks, 1978) or through criterion referenced tests such as the Quality of Upper Extremity Skills Test (QUEST) (DeMatteo et al., 1993).

Object Manipulation

A child's range of grasp patterns can be documented by observing the manipulation of objects of different sizes and shapes such as the ability to display a pincer grasp. Object release can be examined by asking the child to "let go" of an object while the wrist is stabilized manually or with a splint. If a child cannot engage the finger extensors when wrist motion is restricted, they may "shake" the object out of the hand. Stacking blocks, often used in developmental tests, incorporates graded grasp and release.

The fine-motor section of developmental assessments may be used to formally assess manipulation skills of infants and young children (see Table 4). However, results from developmental tests should be interpreted carefully, since the sensitivity of the instrument will vary depending on age and test component (Law et al., 1997). Law and colleagues (1997) used the Peabody Developmental Motor Scales (PDMS-FM) and the Quality of Upper Extremity Skills Test (Quest) to develop growth curves for the development of hand function in children with cerebral palsy. This study highlights how hand function develops differently in this population and how the rate of change is not constant from one to six years of age.

For older children, Sollerman's Grip Test is a tool that rates the range and quality of prehension patterns used to handle objects on a 4-point scale (Sollerman, 1984). Although the test is not very sensitive to small qualitative changes in prehension, it can be used to document the existence of select patterns. Formal tests enhance the quantitative nature of an evaluation, yet it is important to also examine qualitative issues such as movement efficiency.

If a child needs two hands to manipulate objects it may indicate that they have difficulty with *in-hand manipulation* or handling objects with one hand. All three components of in-hand manipulation (translation, shift and rotation) can be tested by placing a crayon or pencil in the palm of a child's hand and asking them to move the crayon or pencil to the fingers (translation), then position it to draw (shift). Rotation can be assessed by asking a child to color with the crayon's flat side or to erase with a pencil. For children with joint contractures or poor muscle activation, in-hand manipulation may be extremely difficult.

Impairments

This level involves the identification of intrinsic constraints to prehension such as impairments in cognition, vision or perception, musculoskeletal components or sensibility. Table 5 lists examples of assessments at the level of impairment.

Cognition

Cognition can be formally assessed using developmental assessments such as the Bayley Scales of Infant Development®, 2nd Ed (BSID-II) (Bayley, 1993) or the Miller Assessment for Preschoolers™ (MAP™) (Miller, 1988) (see Table 4). Because performance is influenced by multiple factors including attention and context, the results should be interpreted carefully (Law et al., 1997). Screening for attentional abilities can be done by monitoring visual regard during object play in infants or by tracking the amount of time a child spends on selective tasks. An overview of cognition and prehension can be found in a chapter by Exner and Henderson (1995).

Motor skills can also provide insight into cognitive and perceptual abilities (Adolph, 1995; Bushnell & Boudreau, 1993). Adolph and colleagues (Adolph, 1995, 2000; Adolph et al., 1993) examined *problem solving* and the perception of *affordances* in infants and toddlers as they learned to ascend and descend slopes and reach over safe and risky gaps. An affordance is the fit or the reciprocal relationship between the environment and the performer used to execute functional tasks (Gibson, 1979). The findings suggest that an infant's approach to motor tasks and ability to "figure out" motor problems are based on perceptual cues and an awareness of capabilities such as postural stability.

Vision

Tests of visual regard and tracking attempt to elicit localization and fixation on near or far, stationary or moving targets through the vertical, horizontal and diagonal planes. Term infants can fixate at or within a short time of birth (Simons, 1993). By two-months of age, visual tracking can be elicited (Casaer & Lagae, 1991). In older infants and children, a functional visual assessment may expand to include tests of visual acuity, binocular fusion, and visual attention (Cavallini et al., 2002; Morale et al., 2002; Richards & Cronise, 2000; Rose et al., 1999).

Impairments in visual perception are often subtle and cannot be easily assessed in infancy. One way to assess perception and problem solving in an infant new to crawling would be to place a familiar object (e.g., bottle) in an atypical position (e.g., upside down) and entice the infant to retrieve it. The motor solution to this task can give the therapist insight into the infant's problem-solving capabilities and visual perceptual skills (e.g., Do they seem to recognize the object and pursue it immediately? What prehensile skills do they employ to retrieve the toy?).

Standardized tests of visual-perception can be helpful when evaluating children. However, the reader is cautioned that many visuo-perceptual tests evaluate two-dimensional (2-D), not three-dimensional (3-D), ability. Because these tests can be misleading it is important to follow-up with functional tests or with observations of perceptual ability in the context of play. If indicated, the therapist should refer the child to other professionals for diagnostic work-up of these problems.

Musculoskeletal Components

Common musculoskeletal tests of range-of-motion and strength are measured through goniometry, manual muscle tests (MMT) and dynamometers (Clarkson & Gilewich, 2000; Fess, 1992; Mathowitz et al., 1986). While muscle activation can be difficult to assess in young infants it is made easier through the elicitation of reflexes such as the Moro. The Active Movement Scale (AMS) (Clarke & Curtis, 1995; Curtis et al., 2002) is another test of muscle function. This 8-point scale was designed for use with infants with brachial plexus birth palsy yet may be useful in other populations and age groups because it tests active unilateral upper limb movement in the gravity-eliminated and against gravity positions and does not require resistive testing.

Sensibility

Passive and active sensibility (stereognosis) tests available for use with older children are listed in Table 5. In young children, it may be sufficient to determine if they feel the touch of an eraser on a finger (passive sensibility) or can identify a known object placed in the hand with vision occluded (active sensibility). A study by Krumlinde-Sundholm and Eliasson (2002) found two-point discrimination, stereognosis of familiar tests and the Pick-up test (with and without vision) to be the most useful in children with neurological impairments.

INTERVENTION:
A TASK ORIENTATED APPROACH

After the assessment is completed, goals and objectives should be established and the method of intervention determined based on collaboration between the family and the therapist (Dunn, 1994). Informal assessment of the key issues continues throughout the intervention period. The types of intervention applicable to prehension within a task-oriented approach are:

1. *Enhancement* of resources to prevent secondary impairments
2. *Promotion* of neuromotor strategies in various contexts
3. *Increasing* function through practice or alteration of task demands/context

Because practice of tasks within the context of daily activity and routines is important for motor learning, involving children and families in

planning interventions is important. Table 7 provides sample intervention strategies from a task-oriented approach for three conditions: Erb's
palsy, arthrogryposis and hemiplegic cerebral palsy.

Enhancement of Resources

Cognition

Cognitive issues of *attention and simple problem solving* are often
obstacles to early skill development regardless of the underlying pathology. Methods to promote attention include reducing distractions

TABLE 7. Sample Intervention Strategies for 3 Conditions Using a Task-Oriented Approach

	Increasing Function	Enhancing Motor Strategies	Enhancing Resources
3-month-old with Erb's palsy	• Increase opportunities for exploration & upper limb movement • Provide support in developmentally appropriate positions such as prone prop with chest roll to support shoulder, alternate right & left sidelying to allow bimanual play & ease shoulder motion	• Increase fixation & following into neglected visual field • Promote unimanual & bimanual flapping & reach to grasp in gravity eliminated & against gravity planes • Provide active assistive movement to increase bimanual awareness & hand play • Encourage lower limb reaching to enhance exploration skills & adaptability	• Place & hold strategies for shoulder, elbow & forearm • Passive range-of-motion (PROM) of GH joint with scapula stabilized • Support arm in external rotation (if tolerated) • Shoulder straps into ER, elbow splints for extension & forearm supination splints as needed • May need microsurgery
2-year-old with Arthrogryposis	• Provide opportunities for exploration of environment & objects • Alter task demands & context to increase ADL & play skills by adapting environment & providing adaptive equipment early (e.g., built-up handles, arm trough for self feeding, switch toys) • Use splints to enhance use of arms & hands	• Set-up environment for unimanual & bimanual reach to grasp in various positions • Provide with bimanual & unimanual manipulative toys & switch toys to promote development of motor strategies • Provide opportunity to explore the environment & objects with lower limbs if they have greater leg strength & range-of-motion	• Place & hold strategies for upper limb • Frequent Passive ROM of all upper limb joints • Alter arm posture at rest (e.g., use tray or table to support in shoulder flexion) • Hand, wrist or elbow splints may be needed to maintain or increase PROM • May need surgical intervention such as joint releases or joint fusions
7-year-old with hemiplegic cerebral palsy	• Increase demand for bimanual performance (e.g., carrying lunch tray, holding bowl while stirring cookie batter) • Consider practice schedules for ADL & play tasks to enhance retention & transfer • Adapt environment to enhance success (e.g., lightweight, shorter baseball bat)	• Play reach to grasp games in multiple areas of the workspace to increase repertoire of motor strategies • Promote bimanual usage or have the non-involved limb perform tasks first to enhance performance in the involved limb • Provide with challenging bimanual manipulative tasks to encourage problem solving	• Theraband for upper limb strengthening • Theraputty, play-doh, legos to increase hand strength • Frequent PROM • Sensory re-education • Hand, wrist or elbow splints as needed • May benefit from surgical or medical intervention such as tendon transfers or Botox • Address visual perception if needed

and allowing the child to choose activities during treatment sessions, incorporating clinical goals into the task of choice. Problem solving could be encouraged through trial and error learning or requiring simple yet independent solutions to movement problems. For example, one could place a favorite toy behind a chair and ask an infant to retrieve it. The infant's solution may involve: (1) crawling through the chair legs to reach and grasp the toy with the non-involved hand, or (2) pulling to stand and cruising around the chair to reach and grasp the toy with the involved hand while the non-involved hand holds the chair for balance.

The reader is referred to other sources for ideas on cognitive rehabilitation pertinent to prehensile skill development in infants and children (e.g., Exner & Henderson, 1995).

Vision

Exercises that train fixation and visual following have been found to be effective at improving upper limb control in adults with neural disorders and enhancing saccadic control in children with dyslexia (Fischer & Hartnegg, 2000; Herdman, 1999). Techniques used for adults (Shumway-Cook & Woollacott, 2001) may be modified for use with infants and children. Setting up the environment with different challenges, then upgrading or downgrading depending on performance is one way to address perceptual issues. For example, to address a "figure-ground" impairment the clinician could initially ask a child to find a button in a box of coins. To increase the complexity, they could ask the child to find the quarters among a box of nickels.

Musculoskeletal Components

Musculoskeletal impairments such as joint or muscle contractures are best addressed with passive range-of-motion (PROM), splinting or serial casting (Cusick, 1988). For minimal impairments periodic PROM may be sufficient. Self-stretching, achieved by moving through an obstacle course in prone or donning a T-shirt over the head, works well for some children. However, a *low-load prolonged stretch* in the form of casts or splints is the best conservative way of increasing PROM (Fess & McCollum, 1998; Nuismer et al., 1997). Smith and Drennan (2002) studied the effect of passive stretching, serial casting and orthotics on wrist position and function in infants with arthrogryposis. At 6-year follow-up, the greatest gain in wrist motion occurred at the first cast session and the largest improvement in function was displayed by infants with distal arthrogryposis. Overall, early treatment for contractures was most effective.

Since infants cannot readily follow commands, problems in muscle strength or imbalance should be incorporated into gross motor play, employing gravity and body parts as forms of resistance. Environmental set-up, playing games such as "Simon Says" or wheel-barrow races for upper limb weight bearing are popular options. To strengthen hands, "play-doh," "theraputty," or the construction of "Lego" projects are often used. Splints or straps may encourage isolation of muscle groups and prevent undesired movement, as seen in Figure 3, used to isolate the elbow flexors.

FIGURE 3. This strap is used to block shoulder abduction in an attempt to isolate active elbow flexion against gravity.

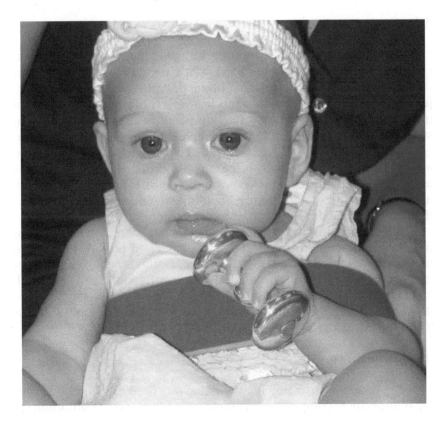

Sensibility

Sensory re-education is an effective technique (Daniele & Aquado, 2003; Rosen & Lundborg, 2003) that requires attention and memory (Dellon & Mackinnon, 1991; Ozkan et al., 2001; Zeuner et al., 2002), thus, should be tailored to a child's cognitive capabilities. Ideally, sensory re-education focuses on passive (externally placed stimuli) and active sensibility (individual moves to obtain sensory stimuli) and protective strategies. Passive sensibility can be promoted with massage and texture discrimination. Active sensibility can be addressed through "hide and seek" object recognition games in rice or macaroni. The reader is referred to guidelines on sensory re-education for further details (Callahan, 2002; Bell-Krotoski, 1993; Byl & McKenzie, 2000).

Improving Neuromotor Strategies for Prehension

Adaptation

The exhibition of variable motor responses requires the inherent capacity to adapt (Ulrich et al., 1997). With a wide repertoire of motor strategies to accomplish a task, an infant or child should be able to adjust their movement(s) to constraints in a variety of contexts. Successful intervention requires the identification of intrinsic and extrinsic constraints unique to each child. For example, children who have insufficient postural control or gross motor skill for prehension may need assistance with exploration by bringing objects to them or vice versa (in addition to methods to improve postural control). The challenge is to identify limitations and resources including the degree of adaptability, then facilitate the development of motor solutions.

Young infants may be capable of object interaction with the hands or feet before the onset of reach to grasp behaviors if provided enhanced movement training (Lobo et al., submitted; Galloway et al., 2002). Objects or overhead mobiles explored via arm flapping or lower limb reaching, may aid the formation of object representations and simple problem solving. Training may encourage the development of adaptable play behaviors.

Anticipatory Behaviors

Methods to improve anticipatory behaviors need to incorporate timing of movement components in preparation for a loss in equilibrium (to prevent going off balance), pre-shaping the hand (to securely attain an object or toy) or grading the fingertip forces (to manipulate objects). Because there are many causes for impaired anticipatory behavior, creative treatment planning including structured practice is essential to success. Intervention will likely require some trial and error on the part of the therapist. The key is to require the planning of movements in advance. For example, ball catching is one task that elicits anticipatory postural adjustments and preparatory reach to grasp with the upper limbs. External devices may help elicit anticipatory behaviors. For example, Figure 4 shows a child without active wrist extension, demonstrating sufficient grip formation in anticipation of receipt of a toy after placement in a semi-mobile wrist splint.

FIGURE 4. Splints such as this mobile wrist support may reveal hidden skills such as the activation of anticipatory grip formation to grasp a toy.

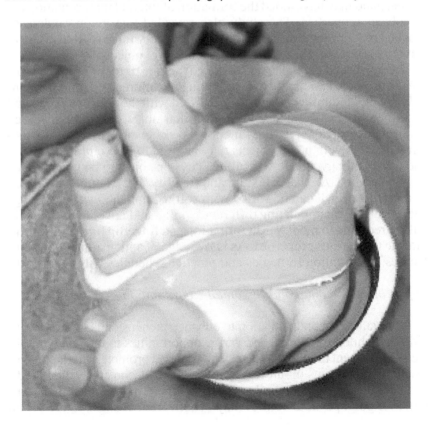

Despite known impairments in anticipatory control, research is only beginning to document how to enhance learning of these behaviors (e.g., Charles et al., 2001; Duff & Gordon, in press; Gordon et al., 1999). Gordon and colleagues (1999) found that children with hemiplegic cerebral palsy displayed anticipatory control during lifts with the involved hand when objects were lifted first with the non-involved hand. They postulated that sensory input gained from lifts with the non-involved hand seemed to aid the formation of internal representations of object properties used for lifts with the involved hand.

Duff and Gordon (in press) recently studied the effect of practice schedules on learning of anticipatory force scaling for familiar and novel objects in children with hemiplegic cerebral palsy. The findings indicate that children with hemiplegia had anticipatory control for lifts of familiar objects with the involved hand. The authors' postulated that extended practice manipulating objects in daily life with the non-involved hand may have aided the formation of internal representations of the object properties. The study also revealed that given random or blocked practice the children learned anticipatory force scaling (as measured by retention) for use during lifts of novel objects.

Therapists and caretakers can take advantage of these research findings to promote anticipatory force scaling in children with unilateral involvement. Unfamiliar objects can be lifted with the non-involved hand first, then the involved. The use of familiar objects with the involved hand can be promoted during functional tasks to ensure success. Structured practice with novel objects may be used to help children acquire and retain anticipatory force scaling. Toys or object to be manipulated should vary in size, shape, texture and fragility. For example, toys such as a small hardball can be varied with soft, compliant ones like a large "nerf" ball. By manipulating different familiar and novel toys, the child will be required to modify grip formation and fingertip forces to accommodate the various properties. As knowledge of anticipatory control increases, intervention strategies and practice schedules will be refined.

Improving Unimanual and Bimanual Coordination

A prevailing recommendation to enhance prehension is to provide infants and children frequent and varied opportunities to interact with objects. Movement training has also been found to promote arm flapping or reaching movements in full-term young infants (Lobo et al., submitted).

The child with upper limb weakness or inefficient movement patterns yet good postural control may benefit from changes in the set-up of the environment or performance demands. For example, changing the target height or location of an object to enhance a new reaching pattern using different muscle groups may expand the repertoire of unimanual or bimanual strategies available to the child. Furthermore, tasks can be altered by changing the timing demands for performance such as asking a child to reach (or throw) as fast or as slow as possible.

Providing the opportunity to explore objects through postural or environmental support is frequently used to enhance reach to grasp skills. Hopkins and Ronnqvist (2002) examined the reaching behaviors of 6-month-olds not yet sitting independently, with and without pelvic and upper leg support. They found head stabilization increased and reaches were smoother when the infants were supported in a chair, providing evidence that infants with motor involvement and inadequate postural control benefit from seating devices that stabilize the trunk. Likewise, children with poor head and neck control may need an adaptive device to provide upright head support promoting visual/spatial orientation in the vertical plane. External postural support may increase the child's tolerance for reaching and grasping activities and so indirectly increase the amount of practice time. As the postural control of the child improves, supports can be removed.

Improving Object Manipulation

As prehension patterns expand and skill at in-hand manipulation increases, dexterity improves. As previously stated, frequent practice time using the hand(s) in various play and functional activities will increase neural representations of object properties which can be used for anticipatory scaling of fingertip forces (Charles et al., 2001). Practice molding resistive fine-motor materials such as clay or cookie-dough can also increase strength of intrinsic hand muscles. Visual-constructive fine-motor tasks place demands on perceptual and problem-solving resources while challenging manipulative skill. Success with simple manipulative tasks (e.g., dialing a toy phone with one hand and holding the handle with the other) may lead to success with more complex tasks (building complex 3-D Lego designs from a 2-D picture).

Structuring Practice

Frequent practice and repetition of activities aids retention of prehensile ability by helping the child attain the general form of the behavior then refining skill. Constructing the infant or child's environment to provide numerous opportunities to practice developing prehension using the involved limb(s) may enhance the likelihood of a limb being used more consistently. Sample modes of practice organization include: generalized or task-related practice, massed versus distributed practice and random or blocked practice.

A study of generalized and task related movement experiences has revealed that toy contact with the feet or hands can be enhanced following training in 8-12 week old infants (Lobo et al., submitted). The authors found that generalized movement experiences resulted in greater foot to toy contacts and task related experiences resulted in greater hand to toy contacts. These findings can be expanded to infants with disabling conditions. The provision of early movement training may help raise interest in exploratory play and serve to expand abilities.

Massed practice involves greater practice time than rest. Distributed practice incorporates greater rest time thus practice is spread out. Constraint-induced therapy (CIT) is a form of massed practice that uses shaping to overcome learned disuse (Taub, 1993). In adults with hemiplegia, the involved arm is constrained in some manner (e.g., sling or splint) forcing the individual to use the involved limb for functional tasks. While the results suggest positive effects, the efficacy of this approach based on outcomes measured by the Motor Activity Log, the Jebsen-Taylor Test of Hand Function and the Wolf Motor Function Test are not conclusive (Charles et al., 2001; Taub & Wolf, 1997). Given this evidence, therapists are recommended to proceed with caution as they implement CIT intervention programs. At the outset, families should be made aware of research findings and the possibility that the effects may range from minimal to broad.

Practice can be arranged in a random or blocked order. A random schedule involves the practice of different task variations on successive trials. In a blocked schedule, one task variation is practiced repeatedly followed by a different one. In adults, blocked practice during training leads to better task performance than random (Gabriele et al., 1987; Lee & Magill, 1983; Shea & Morgan, 1979). Yet, random practice results in better learning as measured by retention or transfer tests. Children or low-skilled performers may learn motor skills best under blocked or serial practice (blocked then random practice) (Del Rey et al., 1983; Herbert et al., 1996; Pigott & Shapiro, 1984; Pinto-Zipp & Gentile, 1995). Yet, Pollock and Lee (1997) found children did better on retention and transfer of a ballistic aiming task after random practice. Findings in clinical groups are mixed (e.g., Duff & Gordon, in press; Hanlon, 1996; Valvano & Newell, 1998).

Because the number of trials (Shea et al., 1990) and level of experience (Wulf & Shea, 2002) influences skill learning, the amount of practice needs to be long enough to enhance retention or transfer. Given the evidence, for complex tasks, such as in-hand manipulation of different sized objects, a child with prehensile dysfunction may begin with blocked practice then progress to serial or random practice. Conversely, random practice may be best for less complex tasks, such as simple grasp and release of objects into various-sized containers, in a child who displays gross grasp function. Regardless of the type, the amount of practice should involve enough trials to enhance learning (more than one treatment session). Despite the recommendations, more research on the effect of different training regimes is warranted.

Altering Task Demands and Context

If a limb is capable of useful prehension the infant or child will likely employ it for function. Intervention may simply involve altering the task demands by changing the location of objects or altering the size and resistance of toys to increase participation and promote the development of varied neuromotor strategies. Furthermore, if a child can begin to meet varied task demands or adjust to modifications in context, prehensile function can expand.

Adaptive equipment for activities of daily living and play or splints can help reduce task demands thus enhance performance. Equipment such as a buttonhook or universal cuff to hold utensils can help some children gain function and improve confidence. Switch toys can help children with minimal hand function engage in age-appropriate play activities. Splints can provide the right amount of limb support to enhance prehension (see Figure 4). Decisions made regarding changes in task demands, adaptive equipment or splints need to be individualized.

CONCLUSION

Increased knowledge of prehension development in infants and children with neuromuscular and musculoskeletal impairments has direct implications for interventions aimed at enhancing functional behavior. While some studies provide solid evidence that intervention for infants and young children is effective in improving postural control and prehensile skill (e.g., Case-Smith, 1996, 2000; Hadders-Algra et al., 1996; Hirschel et al., 1990) others do not (Law et al., 1997). Therefore, further research is needed to identify optimal methods of intervention and practice schedules. In addition, more information is needed on whether early experience or training can prevent disuse or ineffective prehensile strategies from developing. Furthermore, because some infants and children successfully adapt to their functional limitations, examination of how these solutions to prehensile problems are derived and contribute to overall function is warranted. For now, it is incumbent on the therapist to understand and recognize that neuromotor strategies influence the development of prehension and to integrate this knowledge into assessment and intervention. With attention to neuromotor strategies, as well as impairments and function, the prehensile behaviors of infants and children with congenital or acquired deficiencies may be expanded.

REFERENCES

Adolph, K. E. (1995, August). Psychophysical assessment of toddler's ability to cope with slopes. *Journal of Experimental Psychology, Human Perception and Performance, 21* (4), 734-750.

Adolph, K. E. (2000). Specificity of learning: Why infants fall over a veritable cliff. *Psychological Science: A Journal of the American Psychological Society/APS, 11*(4), 290-295.

Adolph, K. E., Eppler, M. A., & Gibson, E. J. (1993, August). Crawling versus walking infants' perception of affordances for locomotion over sloping surfaces. *Child Development, 64*(4), 1158-1174.

Amiel-Tison, C., & Grenier, A. (1983). Expression of Liberated Motor Activity (LMA) following manual immobilization (pp. 87-109). In C. Amiel-Tison, & A. Grenier (Eds.), *Neurological Evaluation of the Newborn and the Infant.* English translation and adaptation by J. J. Steichen, P. Steichen-Asch, & C. P. Braun. New York: Masson. (Original work published 1980).

Amundson, S. (1995). *Evaluation Tool of Children's Handwriting (ETCH).* Homer, AL: O.T. Kids.

Angulo-Kinzler, R. M., Ulrich, B., & Thelen, E. (2002). Three-month-old infants can select specific leg motor solutions. *Motor Control, 6*(1), 52-68.

Ayres, A. J. (1989). *Sensory Integration and Praxis Test.* Torrence, CA: Sensory Integration International.

Bayley, N. (1993). *Bayley Scales of Infant Development (2nd ed.).* New York: The Psychological Corporation.

Beery, K. E. (1997). *The Beery-Butenika Test of Visual-Motor Integration* (4th Revision). Cleveland: Modern Curriculum Press.

Bell-Krotoski, J., Weinstein, S., & Weinstein, C. (1993). Testing sensibility, including touch-pressure, two-point discrimination, point localization, and vibration. *Journal of Hand Therapy, 2,* 114-123.

Benbow, M. (1991). *Loops and Other Groups: A Kinesthetic Writing System.* Instructors's Edition. Randolph, NJ: OT Ideas Inc.

Benbow, M. (1995). *Observation of Hand Skills in the K-1 Child* (Unit 4). Rockville, MD: American Occupational Therapy Association.

Bennett, K. M., & Lemon, R. N. (1996). Corticomotorneuronal contribution to the fractionation of muscle activity during precision grip in the monkey. *Journal of Neurophysiology, 75*(5), 1826-1842.

Susan V. Duff and Jeanne Charles *163*

Bertenthal, B., & Hofsten, C. von. (1998). Eye, head and trunk control: The foundation for manual development. *Neuroscience and Biobehavioral Reviews*, 22(4), 515-20.

Bohannon, R. W., & Smith, M. B. (1987). Inter-rater reliability of a modified Ashworth scale of muscle spasticity. *Physical Therapy, 67*, 206-207.

Brown, J. K., Rensburg, Van E., Walsh, G., Lakie, M., & Wright, G. W. (1987). A neurological study of hand function of hemiplegic children. *Developmental Medicine & Child Neurology, 38*, 951-964.

Brunicks, R. H. (1978). *Bruininks-Oseretsky Test of Motor Proficiency*. Circle Pine, MN: American Guidance Service.

Bushnell, E. W., & Boudreau, J. P. (1993, August). Motor development and the mind: The potential role of motor abilities as a determinant of aspects of perceptual development. *Child Development, 64*(4), 1005-1021.

Byl, N. N., & McKenzie, A. (2000). Treatment effectiveness for patients with a history of repetitive hand use and focal hand dystonia: A planned prospective follow-up study. *Journal of Hand Therapy, 13*(4), 289-301.

Callahan, A. D. (2002). Sensibility assessment for nerve lesions–in continuity and nerve lacerations. In E. J. Mackin, A. D. Callahan, Skirven, T. M., L. S. Schneider, & A. L. Osterman (Eds.), *Hunter-Mackin-Callahan Rehabilitation of the Hand and Upper Extremity* (5th ed., pp. 214-239). Philadelphia: Mosby.

Casaer, P., & Lagae, L. (1991). Age specific approach to neurological assessment in the first year of life. *Acta Paediatrica Japan, 33*, 125-138.

Case-Smith, J. (2000). Effects of occupational therapy services on fine motor and functional performance in preschool children. *American Journal of Occupational Therapy, 54*(4), 372-380.

Case-Smith, J. (1996). Fine motor outcomes in preschool children who receive occupational therapy services. *American Journal of Occupational Therapy, 50*(1), 52-61.

Cavallini, A., Fazzi, E., Viviani, V., Astori, M. G., Zaverio, S., Bianchi, P. E., & Lanzi, G. (2002, Apr-June). Visual acuity in the first two years of life in healthy term newborns: An experience with the teller acuity cards. *Functional Neurology, 17*(2), 87-92.

Charles, J. (1999). Constraint-induced therapy in children with hemiplegic cerebral palsy. Poster presention made at *The Combined Sections Meeting of The American Physical Therapy Association*.

Charles, J., Lavender, G., & Gordon, A. M. (2001). Constraint induced therapy in children with hemiplegic cerebral palsy. *Pediatric Physical Therapy, 13*(2), 68-76.

Clarke, H. M., & Curtis, C. G. (1995, November). An approach to obstetrical brachial plexus injuries. *Hand Clinics, 11*(4), 563-580.

Clarkson, H. M., & Gilewich, G. B. (2000). *Musculoskeletal Assessment: Joint Range-of-Motion and Manual Muscle Strength* (2nd ed.). Baltimore MD: Williams & Wilkins.

Cohen, E., Boettcher, K., Maher, T., Phillips, A., Terrel, L., Nixon-Cave, K., & Shephard, K. (1999). Evaluation of the Peabody Developmental Gross Motor Scales for young children of African American and Hispanic ethnic backgrounds. *Pediatric Physical Therapy, 11*(4), 191-204.

Colarusso, R. P., & Hammill, D. D. (1996). *Motor Free Visual Perceptual Test-Revised*. Los Angeles, CA: Western Psychological Services.

Corbetta, D., & Bojczyk, K. E. (2002). Infants return to two-handed reaching when they are learning to walk. *Journal of Motor Behavior, 34*(1), 83-95.

Corbetta, D., & Thelen, E. (1996). The developmental orgins of bimanual coordination: A dynamic perspective. *Journal of Experimental Psychology: Human Perception and Performance, 22* (2), 502-522.

Coster, W., Deeney, T., Haltiwanger, J., & Haley, S. (1998). *School Function Assessment (SFA)*. San Antonio: The Psychological Corporation of Harcourt Brace & Co.

Curtis, C., Stephens, D., Clarke, H. M., & Andrews, D. (2002). The active movement scale: An evaluative tool for infants with obstetrical brachial plexus palsy. *Journal of Hand Surgery, 7*(3), 470-478.

Cusick, B. D. (1988, December) Splints and casts. Managing foot deformity in children with neuromotor disorders. *Physical Therapy, 68*(12), 1903-1912.

Daniele, H. R., & Aguado, L. (2003, February). Early compensatory sensory re-education. *Journal of Reconstructive Microsurgery, 19*(2), 107-110.

D'Elia, A., Pighetti, M., Moccia, G., & Santangelo, N. (2001). Spontaneous motor activity in normal fetuses. *Early Human Development, 65*(2), 139-147.

Dellon, A. L. (1981). *Evaluation of Sensibility and Reeducation of Sensation in the Hand*. Baltimore: Williams & Wilkins.

Dellon, A. L., & Mackinnon, S. E. (1991). Results of posterior tibial nerve grafting at the ankle. *Journal of Reconstructive Microsurgery, 7*(2), 81-83.

DelRay, P., Whitehurst, M., Wughalter, E., & Barnwell, J. (1983). Contextual interference and experience in acquisition and transfer. *Perceptual Motor Skills, 57,* 241-242.

DeMatteo, C., Law, M., Russell, D., Pollock, N., Rosenbaum, P., & Walter, S. (1993). The reliability and validity of the Quality of Upper Extremity Skills Test. *Physical & Occupational Therapy in Pediatrics, 13,* 1-18.

Depoy, E., & Gitlow, L. (2001). A model of evidence-based practice for Occupational Therapy In L. W. Pedretti, & W. B. Early (Eds.), *Occupational Therapy: Practice Skills for Physical Dysfunction* (5th ed., pp. 58-68). Philadelphia: Mosby.

DeVries, H. I., Wimmers, R. H., Ververs, I. A., Hopkins, B., Savelsbergh, G. J. & Geijn, H. P. van (2001). Fetal handedness and head position preference: A developmental study. *Developmental Psychobiology, 39*(3), 171-178.

DiPietro, J. A., Bornstein, M. H., Costigan, K A., Pressman, E. K., Hahn, C. S., Painter, K., Smith, B. A., & Yi, L. J. (2002). What does fetal movement predict about behavior during the first two years of life? *Developmental Psychobiology, 40*(4), 358-371.

Duff, S. V, Shumway-Cook, A., & Woollacott, M. (2001). Clinical management of reach, grasp and manipulation disorders. In A. Shumway-Cook & M. Woollacott (Eds.), *Motor Control: Theory and Practical Applications* (2nd ed., pp. 517-560). Baltimore: Lippincott Williams & Wilkins.

Duff, S. V. (2002). Prehension. In D. J. Cech, & S. Martin (Eds.), *Functional Movement Development Across the Lifespan* (2nd ed., pp. 517-560). Philadelphia: W. B Saunders.

Duff, S. V., & Gordon, A. M. (in press). Learning of grasp control in children with hemiplegic cerebral palsy. *Developmental Medicine & Child Neurology*.

Dunn, W., Brown, C., & McGuigan, A. (1994). The ecology of human performance: A framework for considering the effect of context. *American Journal of Occupational Therapy, 48*, 595-607.

Eliasson, A. C., & Gordon, A. M. (2000). Impaired force coordination during object release in children with hemiplegic cerebral palsy. *Developmental Medicine & Child Neurology, 42*(4), 28-34.

Eliasson, A. C., Gordon, A. M., & Forssberg, H. (1991). Basic coordination of manipulative forces in children with cerebral palsy. *Developmental Medicine & Child Neurology, 33*, 661-670.

Eliasson, A. C., Gordon, A. M., & Forssberg, H. (1992). Impaired anticipatory control of isometric forces during grasping by children with cerebral palsy. *Developmental Medicine & Child Neurology, 34*, 216-225.

Eliasson, A. C., Gordon, A. M., & Forssberg, H. (1995). Tactile control of isometric fingertip forces during grasping in children with cerebral palsy. *Developmental Medicine & Child Neurology, 7*, 72-84.

Erhardt, R. P. (1971). *Developmental Hand Dysfunction: Theory, Assessment, and Treatment.* Laurel, MD: RAMSCO.

Erhardt, R. P. (1982). *Developmental Hand Dysfunction: Theory, Assessment, and Treatment.* (pp. 9-43). Laurel, MD: RAMSCO.

Exner, C. (1993). Assessment of manipulation skills. Presented at the Annual American Occupational Therapy Conference. Seattle, WA.

Exner, C. (1990). The zone of proximal development in in-hand manipulation skills of nondysfunctional 3 and 4 year old children. *American Journal of Occupational Therapy, 44*(10), 884-891.

Exner, C. & Henderson, A. (1995). Cognition and motor skill. In Henderson, A., & Pehoski, C. (Eds.), *Hand Function in the Child: Foundations for Remediation* (pp. 93-110). Boston: Mosby.

Fallang, B., Saugstad, O. D., & Hadders-Algra, M. (2000). Goal directed reaching and postural control in supine position in healthy infants. *Behavioral Brain Research, 115*(1), 9-18.

Fess, E. E. (1992). Grip strength. In J. Cassanova (Ed.), *Clinical Assessment Recommendations* (2nd ed., pp. 41-45). American Society of Hand Therapists.

Fess, E. E., & McCollum, M. (1998, April-June). The influence of splinting on healing tissues. *Journal of Hand Therapy, 11*(2), 157-161.

Fischer, B., & Hartnegg, K. (2000). Effects of visual training on saccade control in dyslexia. *Perception, 29*(5), 531-542.

Folio, R. M., & Fewell, R. R. (1983). *Peabody Developmental Motor Scales.* Allen, TX: DLM Teaching Resources.

Forssberg, H., Eliasson, A. C., Kinoshita, H., Johansson, R. S., & Westling, G. (1991). Development of human precision grip: Basic coordination of force. *Experimental Brain Research, 85*, 451-457.

Forssberg, H., Eliasson, A. C., Kinoshita, H., Johansson, R. S., & Westling, G. (1995). Development of human precision grip IV: Tactile adaptation of isometric finger forces to the frictional condition. *Experimental Brain Research, 104*, 323-330.

Forssberg, H., Kinoshita, H., Eliasson, A. C., Johansson, R. S., Westling, G., & Gordon, A. M. (1992). Development of human precision grip II. Anticipatory control of isometric forces targeted for object's weight. *Experimental Brain Research, 90*, 393-398.

Gabriele, T. E., Hall, C. R., & Buckolz, E. E. (1987). Practice schedule effects on the acquisition and retention of a motor skill. *Human Movement Science, 6*, 1-16.

Galloway, J. C., & Thelen, E. (in press). Feet first: Object exploration in human infants. *Infant Behavior and Development.*

Galloway, J., Heathcock, J., Bhat, A., & Lobo, M. (2002, April). Feet reaching: The interaction of experience and ability. Abstract from International Conference on Infant Studies. Toronto, Canada.

Gardner, M. F. (1996). *Test of Visual-Perceptual Skills (n-m) Revised.* Psychological and Educational Publications.

Gentile, A. M. (1998). Implicit and explicit learning processes during acquisition of functional skills. *Scandanavian Journal of Occupational Therapy, 5*, 7-16.

Gibson, J. J. (1979). *The Ecological Approach to Visual Perception.* Boston: Houghton Mifflin.

Goodale, M. A., Meenan, J. P., Bulthoff, H. H., Nicolle, D. A., Murphy, K.S., & Raciecot, C. I. (1994). Separate neuronal pathways for the visual analysis of object shape in perception and prehension. *Current Biology, 4*, 604-610.

Gordon, A. M., Charles, J., & Duff, S. V. (1999). Fingertip forces during object manipulation in children with hemiplegic cerebral palsy II: Bilateral coordination. *Developmental Medicine & Child Neurology, 41*,176-185.

Gordon, A. M., & Duff, S. V. (1999a). Fingertip forces during object manipulation in children with hemiplegic cerebral palsy I: Anticipatory scaling. *Developmental Medicine & Child Neurology, 41*, 166-175.

Gordon, A. M., & Duff, S. V. (1999b). Relation between clinical measures and fine manipulative control in children with hemiplegic cerebral palsy. *Developmental Medicine & Child Neurology, 41*, 586-591.

Gordon, A. M., Lewis, S. R., Eliasson, A. C., & Duff, S. V. (2003). Object release under varying task constraints in children with hemiplegic cerebral palsy. *Developmental Medicine & Child Neurology, 45*, 240-248.

Gordon, A. M., Westling, G., Cole, K. J., & Johansson, R. S. (1993). Memory representations underlying motor commands used during manipulation of common and novel objects. *Journal of Neurophysiology, 69*, 1789-1796.

Hadders-Algra, M., Van der Fits, I. B., Stremmelaar, E. F., & Touwen, B. C. (1999). Development of postural adjustments during reaching in infants with CP. *Developmental Medicine & Child Neurology, 41*(11), 766-776.

Hahn, G. (1985, April). Arthrogryposis. Pediatric review and habilitative aspects. *Clinical Orthopedics*, (194), 104-114.

Haley, S. M., Coster, W. J., Ludlow, L. H., Haltiwanger, J. T., & Andrellos, P. J. (1992). *Pediatric Evaluation of Disability Inventory (PEDI).* Boston: New England Medical Center Hospitals.

Hanlon, R. E. (1996). Motor learning following unilateral stroke. *Archives of Physical Medicine and Rehabilitation, 77*, 811-815.

Hanna, S. E., Law, M. C., Rosenbaum, P. L., King, G. A., Walter, S. D., Pollock, N., & Russell, D. J. (2003). Development of hand function among children with cerebral palsy: Growth curve analysis for ages 16-70 months. *Developmental Medicine & Child Neurology, 45*, 418-455.

Herbert, E. P., Landin, D., & Solmon, M. A. (1996). Practice schedule effects on the performance and learning of low- and high-skilled students: An applied study. *Research Quarterly for Exercise and Sport, 67*, 52-58.

Herdman, S. J. (1999).*Vestibular Rehabilitation.* Philadelphia, PA: FA Davis.

Hirschel, A., Pehoski, C., & Coryell, J. (1990). Environmental support and the development of grasp in infants. *American Journal of Occupational Therapy, 44*(8), 721-727.

Hofsten, C. von (1997). On the early development of predictive abilities. In C. Dent-Read, & P. Zukow-Goldring (Eds.), *Evolving Explanations of Development* (pp. 163-194). Washington, D.C.: American Psychological Association.

Hofsten, C. von, & Fazel-Zandy, S. (1984). Development of visually guided hand orientation in reaching. *Journal of Experimental Child Psychology, 38*(2), 208-219.

Hofsten, C. von, & Lindhagen, K. (1979). Observation on the development of reaching for moving objects. *Journal of Experimental Child Psychology, 28*, 158-173.

Hofsten C. von, & Ronnqvist, L. (1988). Preparation for grasping an object: A developmental study. *Journal of Experimental Psychology: Human Perception and Performance, 14*, 610-621.

Hofsten, C. von, & Ronnqvist, L. (1993). The structuring of neonatal arm movements. *Child Development, 64*(4), 1046-1057.

Hofsten, C. von, & Rosander, K. (1997). Development of smooth pursuit tracking in young infants. *Vision Research, 37*(13), 1799-1810.

Hopkins, B. & Ronnqvist, L. (2002). Facilitating postural control: Effects on the reaching behavior of 6 month-old infants. *Developmental Psychobiology, 40*(2), 168-82.

Jackobson, L. S., & Goodale, M. A. (1991). Factors affecting higher-order movement planning: A kinematic analysis of human prehension. *Experimental Brain Research, 86*, 199-208.

Jeannerod, M. (1981). Intersegmental coordination during reaching at natural visual objects. In J. Long & A. Baddeley (Eds.), *Attention and Performance IX* (pp. 153-168). Hillsdale: Earlbaum.

Jeannerod, M. (1990). *The Neural and Behavioral Organization of Goal-Directed Movements.* Oxford: Claredon.

Jeannerod, M. (1984). The timing of natural prehension movements. *Journal of Motor Behavior, 16*, 235-254.

Jebsen, R. H., Taylor, N. Trieschmann, R. B., Trotter, M. J., & Howard, L. (1969). An objective and standard test of hand function. *Archives of Physical Medicine & Rehabilitation, 50*, 311-319.

Johansson, R. S. (1996). Sensory control of dexterous manipulation in humans. In A. M. Wing, P. Haggard, & J. Flanagan (Eds.), *Hand and Brain: The Neurophysiology and Psychology of Hand Movements* (pp. 381-414). New York: Academic Press.

Johansson, R. S., & Cole, K. J. (1992). Sensory-motor coordination during grasping and manipulative actions. *Current Opinion in Neurobiology, 2*(6), 815-823.

Johansson, R., & Westling, G. (1984). Factors influencing the force control during precision grip. *Experimental Brain Research, 53*, 277-284.

Johansson, R. S., & Westling, G. (1987). Signals in tactile afferents from the fingers eliciting adaptive motor responses during precision grip. *Experimental Brain Research, 66*, 141-154.

Johansson, R. S., & Westling, G. (1988). Coordinated isometric muscle commands adequately and erroneously programmed for the weight during lifting task with precision grip. *Experimental Brain Research, 71*, 59-71.

Johnson, L. M., Randall, M. J., Reddihough, D. S., Oke, L. E., Byrt, T. A., & Bach, T. M. (1994, November). Development of a clinical assessment of quality of movement for unilateral upper-limb function. *Developmental Medicine & Child Neurology, 36*(11), 965-73

Kawai, M., Savelsbergh, G. J., & Wimmers, R. H. (1999). Newborns spontaneous arm movements are influenced by the environment. *Early Human Development, 54*(1), 15-27.

Konczak, J., & Dichgans, J. (1997). The development toward stereotypic arm kinematics during reaching in the first 3 years of life. *Experimental Brain Research, 117*, 346-354.

Krumlinde-Sundholm, L., & Eliasson, A. C. (2002). Comparing tests of tactile sensibility: Aspects relevant to testing children with spastic hemiplegia. *Developmental Medicine & Child Neurology, 44*(9), 604-612.

Kuhtz-Buschbeck, J. P., Stolze, H., Boczek-Funcke, A., Johnk, K., Boczek-Funcke, A., & Illert, M. (1998a). Development of prehension movements in children: A kinematic study. *Experimental Brain Research, 122*, 424-432.

Kuhtz-Buschbeck, J. P., Stolze, H., Boczek-Funcke, A., Johnk, K., Heinrichs, H., & Illert, M. (1998b). Kinematic analysis of prehension movements in children. *Behavioral Brain Research,* (1-2), 131-141.

Kurjak, A., Vecek, N., Hafner, T., Bozek, T., Funduk-Kurjak, B., & Ujevic, B. (2002). Prenatal diagnosis: What does four-dimensional ultrasound add? *Journal of Perinatal Medicine, 30*(1), 57-62.

Kuypers, H. G. (1978). The motor system and the capacity to execute highly fractionated distal extremity movements. *Electroencephalography and Clinical Neurophysiology, Supplemental,* (34), 429-431.

Lantz, C., Melen, K., & Forssberg, H. (1996). Early infant grasping involves radial fingers. *Developmental Medicine & Child Neurology, 38*, 668-674.

Law, M. C., Russell, D. J., Pollock, N., Rosenbaum, P. L., Walter, S. D., & King, G. A. (1997). A comparison of intensive neurodevelopmental therapy plus casting and a regular occupational therapy program for children with cerebral palsy. *Developmental Medicine & Child Neurology, 39*, 664-670.

Lee, T. D., & Magill, R. A. (1983). The locus of contextual interference in motor-skill acquisition. *Journal of Experimental Psychology: Learning, Memory and Cognition, 9*, 730-746.

Lobo, M. A., Galloway, J. C., & Savelsbergh, G. J. P. (Submitted). The effects of specific and general practice on the development of reaching. Under review in *Child Development*.

Manske, P.R., Rotman, M.B., & Dailey, L.A. (1992). Long-term functional results after pollicization for the congenitally deficient thumb. *Journal of Hand Surgery, 17*, 1064-1072.

Mathiowetz, V., Wiemer, D. M., & Federman, S. M. (1986). Grip and pinch strength norms for 6 to 19 year olds. *American Journal of Occupational Therapy, 40*(10), 705-711.

McCartney, G., & Hepper, P. (1999). Development of lateralized behaviour in the human fetus from 12 to 27 week's gestation. *Developmental Medicine & Child Neurology, 41*(2), 83-86.

Morale, S. E., Jeffrey, B. G., Fawcett, S. L., Stager, D. R., Salomao, S. R., Berezovsky, A., Lapa, M. C., & Birch, E. E. (2002, August). Preschool Worth 4-shape test: Testability, reliability, and validity. *Journal of AAPOS: The official publication of the American Association for Pediatric Ophthalmology and Strabismus/American Association for Pediatric Ophthalmology and Strabismus, 6*(4), 247-251.

Msall, M. E., DiGaudio, K., Duffy, L. C., LaForest, S., Braun, S., & Granger, C. V. (1994, July). WeeFIM. Normative sample of an instrument for tracking functional independence in children. *Clinical Pediatrics (Philadelphia), 33*(7), 431-438.

Nagi, S. Z. (1965). Some conceptual issues in disability and rehabilitation. In: M. D. Sussman (Ed.), *Sociology and Rehabilitation* (pp. 100-113). Washington: American Sociological Association.

Napier, J. R. (1956). The prehensile movement of the human hand. *Journal of Joint Surgery* [Br], *38*, 902-913.

National Center for Medical Rehabilitation Research (NCMRR). (1992). *National Advisory Board for Medical Rehabilitation Research, Draft V Report and Plan for Medical Rehabilitation Research.* Bethesda, MD: National Institutes of Health (NIH).

Newell, K. M., Scully, D.M., McDonald, P.V., & Baillargeon, R. (1989). Task constraints and infant grip configurations. *Developmental Psychobiology, 22*(8), 817-831.

Nuismer, B. A., Ekes, A. M., & Holm, M. B. (1997). The use of low-load prolonged stretch devices in rehabilitation programs in the Pacific northwest. *American Journal of Occupational Therapy, 51*(7), 538-543.

Ozkan, T., Ozer, K., & Gulgonen, A. (2001). Restoration of sensibility in irreparable ulnar and median nerve lesions with use of sensory nerve transfer: Long-term follow-up of 20 cases. *Journal of Hand Surgery, 26*(1), 44-51.

Page, S. J., Sisto, S. A., Levine, P., Johnston, M. V., & Hughes, M. (2001). Modified constraint induced therapy: A randomized feasibility and efficacy study. *Journal of Rehabilitation Research and Development, 38*(5), 583-90.

Palmer, P. M., MacEwen, G. C., Bowen, J. R., & Mathews, P. A. (1985, April). Passive motion therapy for infants with arthrogryposis. *Clinical Orthopedics* (194), 54-59.

Pehoski, C. (1995). Object manipulation in infants and children. In Henderson, A., & Pehoski, C. (Eds.), *Hand Function in the Child: Foundations for Remediation* (pp. 136-153). Boston: Mosby.

Pigott, R. E., & Shapiro, D. C. (1984). Motor schema: The structure of the variability session. *Research Quarterly for Exercise and Sport, 61,* 169-177.

Pinto-Zipp, G., & Gentile, A. M. (1995). Practice schedules in motor learning: Children vs. adults. *Society for Neuroscience Abstracts, 21,* 1620(AQ27).

Pollock, B. J., & Lee, T. D. (1997). Dissociated contextual interference in children and adults. *Perceptual Motor Skills, 84*(3 Pt 1), 851-858.

Ramos, L. E., & Zell, J. P. (2000). Rehabilitation program for children with brachial plexus and peripheral nerve injury. *Seminars in Pediatric Neurology, 7*(1), 52-57.

Randall, M., Carlin, J. B., Chondros, P., & Reddihough, D. (2001, November). Reliability of the Melbourne assessment of unilateral upper limb function. *Developmental Medicine & Child Neurology, 43*(11), 761-767.

Richards, J. E., & Cronise, K. (2000, May-June). Extended visual fixation in the early preschool years: Look duration, heart rate changes, and attentional inertia. *Child Development, 71*(3), 602-20.

Rochat, P. (1992). Self-sitting and reaching in 5- to 8-month-old infants: The impact of posture and its development on eye-hand coordination. *Journal of Motor Behavior, 24*, 210-220.

Rosander, K., & Hofsten, C. von. (2000). Visual-vestibular interaction in early infancy. *Experimental Brain Research, 133*(3), 321-33.

Rose, S. A., Futterweit, L. R., & Jankowski, J. J. (1999, May-June). The relation of affect to attention and learning in infancy. *Child Development, 70*(3), 539-559.

Rosen, B., & Lundborg, G. (2003). Early use of artificial sensibility to improve sensory recovery after repair of the median and ulnar nerve. *Scandinavian Journal of Plastic and Reconstructive Surgery and Hand Surgery, 37*(1), 54-7.

Rovee-Collier, C. K., & Sullivan, M. W. (1980). Organization of infant memory. *Journal of Experimental Psychology, [Human Learning] 6*(6), 798-807.

Schneck, C. M., & Henderson, A. (1990). Descriptive analysis of the developmental progression of grip position for pencil and crayon control in nondysfunctional children. *American Journal of Occupational Therapy, 44*, 893-900.

Shea, C. H., Kohl, R., & Indermill, C. (1990). Contextual interference: Contributions of practice. *Acta Psychologia, 73*, 145-157.

Shea, J. B., & Morgan, R. L. (1979). Contextual interference effects on the acquisition, retention, and transfer of a motor skill. *Journal of Experimental Psychology, 5*(2), 179-187.

Shumway-Cook, A., & Woollacott, M. H. (2001). *Motor Control: Theory and Practical Applications* (2nd ed.). Philadelphia: Lippincott Williams & Wilkins.

Simons, K. (1993). *Early Visual Development, Normal and Abnormal.* New York: Oxford University Press.

Smith, D. W, & Drennan, J. C. (2002). Arthrogryposis wrist deformities: Results of infantile serial casting. *Journal of Pediatric Orthopedics, 22*(1), 44-47.

Sollerman, C. (1984). Assessment of grip function: Evaluation of a new method. Sweden: *MITAB.*

Sparling, J. W., Van Tol, J., & Chescheir, N. C. (1999). Fetal and neonatal hand movement. *Physical Therapy, 79*(1), 24-39.

Spencer, J. P., & Thelen, E. (2000). Spatially specific changes in infant's muscle coactivity as they learn to reach. *Infancy, 1*(3), 275-302.

Steenbergen, B., Hulstijn, W., Lemmens, I. H. L., & Meulenbroek, R. G. J. (1998). The timing of prehensile movements in subjects with cerebral palsy. *Developmental Medicine & Child Neurology, 40*, 108-114.

Sterr, A., Elbert, T., Berthhold, I., Kolbel, S., Rockstroh, B., & Taub, E. (2002). Longer versus shorter daily constraint-induced movement therapy of chronic hemiparesis: An exploratory study. *Archives in Physical Medicine & Rehabilitation, 83*(10), 1374-1377.

Stone, J. H. (1992). Sensibility. In J. Cassanova (Ed.), *Clinical Assessment Recommendations* (2nd ed., pp. 71-84). American Society of Hand Therapists.

Sullivan, M. W., Rovee-Collier, C. K., & Tynes, D. M. (1979). A conditioning analysis of infant long-term memory. *Child Development, 50*(1), 152-162.

Tardieu, C., Lespargot, A., Tabary, C., & Bret, M. D. (1988). For how long must the soleus muscle be stretched each day to prevent contracture? *Developmental Medicine & Child Neurology, 30*(1), 3-10.

Taub, E. (1993). Technique to improve chronic motor deficit after stroke. *Archives in Physical Medicine & Rehabilitation, 74*, 347-354.

Taub, E., & Wolf, S. L. (1997). Constraint-Induction/forced use techniques to facilitate upper extremity use in stroke patients. *Topics in Stroke Rehabilitation, 3*, 38-61.

Taylor, N., Sand, P. L., & Jebsen, R. H. (1973). Evaluation of hand function in children. *Archives in Physical Medicine & Rehabilitation, 54*(3), 129-135.

Thelen, E. (1998). Bernstein's legacy for motor development: How infants learn to reach. In: M. Latash (Ed.), *Progress in Motor Control (vol 1): Bernstein's Traditions in Movement Studies* (pp. 267-288). Champaign, IL: Human Kinetics.

Thelen, E. (1995). Motor development. A new synthesis. *American Psychologist, 50*(2), 79-95.

Thelen, E., Corbetta, D., Kamm, K., Spencer, J. P., Schneider, K., & Zernicke, R. F. (1993). The transition to reaching: Mapping intention and intrinsic dynamics. *Child Development, 64*(4), 1058-1098.

Thelen, E., Corbetta, D., & Spencer, J. P. (1996). Development of reaching during the first year: Role of movement speed. *Journal of Experimental Psychology, Human Perception and Performance, 22*(5), 1059-1076.

Thelen, E., & Spencer, J. P. (1998). Postural control during reaching in young infants: A dynamic systems approach. *Neuroscience and Biobehavioral Reviews, 22*(4), 507-14.

Ulrich, B. D., Ulrich, D. A., Angulo-Kinzler, R., & Chapman, D. D. (1997, March). Sensitivity of infants with and without Down Syndrome to intrinsic dynamics. *Research Quarterly for Exercise and Sport, 68*(1), 10-19.

Utley, A., & Sugden, D. (1998). Interlimb coupling in children with hemiplegic cerebral palsy during reaching and grasping at speed. *Developmental Medicine & Child Neurology, 40*, 396-404.

Valvano, J., & Newell, K. M. (1998). Practice of a precision isometric grip-force task by children with spastic cerebral palsy. *Developmental Medicine & Child Neurology, 40*, 464-473.

Van der Fits, I. B., & Hadders-Algra, M. (1998). The development of postural response patterns during reaching in healthy infants. *Neuroscience and Biobehavioral Reviews, 22*(4), 521-526.

Van der Fits, I. B., Klip, A. W., Van Eykern, L. A., & Hadders-Algra, M. (1999a). Postural adjustments during spontaneous and goal-directed arm movements in the first half year of life. *Behavioral Brain Research, 106*(1-2), 75-90.

Van der Fits, I. B., Otten, E., Klip, A. W., Van Eykern, L. A., & Hadders-Algra, M. (1999b). The development of postural adjustments during reaching in 6- to 18-month-old infants. Evidence for two transitions. *Experimental Brain Research, 126*(4), 517-28.

Waters, P. (1997). Obstetric brachial plexus injuries: Evaluation and management. *Journal of the American Academy of Orthopedic Surgery, 5*(4), 205-214.

WeeFIM System ® Clinical Guide: Version 5.01 Buffalo, NY 14214: University of Buffalo; 1998.

Weinstein, S. (1993, January-March). Fifty years of somatosensory research: From the Semmes-Weinstein monofilaments to the Weinstein Enhanced Sensory Test. *Journal of Hand Therapy, 6*(1), 11-22.

Westling, G., & Johansson, R. S. (1987). Responses in glabrous skin mechanoreceptors during precision grip in humans. *Experimental Brain Research, 66,* 128-140.

Woollacott, M. & Shumway-Cook, A. (1986). The development of the postural and voluntary motor control system in Down's syndrome children. In M. Wade (Ed.), *Motor Skill Acquisition of the Mentally Handicapped: Issues in Research and Training* (pp. 45-71). Amsterdam: Elsevier.

World Health Organization (WHO). (1980). *International Classification of Impairments, Disabilities, and Handicaps.* Geneva, Switzerland: World Health Organization.

Wulf, G., & Shea, C. H. (2002). Principles derived from the study of simple skills do not generalize to complex skill learning. *Psychonomic Bulletin & Review, 9,* 185-211.

Zeuner, K. E., Bara-Jimenez, W., Noguchi, P. S., Goldstein, S. R., Dambrosia, J. M., & Hallet, M. (2002). Sensory training for patients with focal hand dystonia. *Annals in Neurology, 51*(5), 593-598.

Reliability of a Measure
of Muscle Extensibility
in Fullterm and Preterm Newborns

Marybeth Grant Beuttler
Peter M. Leininger
Robert J. Palisano

SUMMARY. *Purpose*: The purpose of this study was to examine the test-retest and inter-rater reliability of a measure of muscle extensibility developed by Tardieu, de la Tour, Bret, and Tardieu (1982) in fullterm and preterm newborns.

Marybeth Grant Beuttler, PT, MS, is Assistant Professor of Physical Therapy, University of Scranton, Scranton, Pennsylvania, and a doctoral candidate at Drexel University, Hahnemann Programs in Rehabilitation Sciences, Philadelphia, Pennsylvania. Peter M. Leininger, MPT, is Assistant Professor of Physical Therapy, University of Scranton, Pennsylvania and a doctoral student at Temple University, Department of Physical Therapy, Philadelphia, Pennsylvania. Robert J. Palisano, PT, ScD, is Professor, Program in Rehabilitation Sciences, Drexel University, Philadelphia, Pennsylvania.

Address correspondence to: Marybeth Grant Beuttler, PT, MS, University of Scranton, 800 Linden Avenue, Scranton, PA 18510 (Email: grantbeuttm2@uofs.edu).

The first author would like to thank Community Medical Center in Scranton, Pennsylvania, neonatologist Dr. J. Delfor Salazar, neonatal staff educator, Karen Caputo, and the nursing staff in the newborn nursery and the NICU.

This project was approved by the Internal Review Board at the University of Scranton and the Executive Committee at Community Medical Center.

[Haworth co-indexing entry note]: "Reliability of a Measure of Muscle Extensibility in Fullterm and Preterm Newborns." Beuttler, Marybeth Grant, Peter M. Leininger, and Robert J. Palisano. Co-published simultaneously in *Physical & Occupational Therapy in Pediatrics* (The Haworth Press, Inc.) Vol. 24, No. 1/2, 2004, pp. 173-186; and: *Movement Sciences: Transfer of Knowledge into Pediatric Therapy Practice* (ed: Robert J. Palisano) The Haworth Press, Inc., 2004, pp. 173-186. Single or multiple copies of this article are available for a fee from The Haworth Document Delivery Service [1-800-HAWORTH, 9:00 a.m. - 5:00 p.m. (EST). E-mail address: docdelivery@haworthpress.com].

Method: Twenty-one fullterm infants and twenty preterm infants were examined by two physical therapists. Each physical therapist measured A_0 (shortened position of the muscle belly and lengthened tendon) and A_{Max} (maximum muscle belly and tendon length) of the gastrocnemius/soleus muscle twice in succession. Reliability was assessed using intraclass correlation coefficients (2,2) and (3,2).

Results: Inter-rater reliability between the two examiners ranged from .86 to .97 and test-retest reliability on the two measures ranged from .91 to .98.

Conclusions: The results suggest that this measure of muscle extensibility is reliable in the gastrocnemius/soleus muscle with fullterm and preterm newborns. Further research is needed to investigate if differences in muscle extensibility are present between fullterm and preterm infants and the relationship between muscle extensibility and active movement. *[Article copies available for a fee from The Haworth Document Delivery Service: 1-800-HAWORTH. E-mail address: <docdelivery@haworthpress.com> Website: <http://www.HaworthPress.com> © 2004 by The Haworth Press, Inc. All rights reserved.]*

KEYWORDS. Preterm infants, motor development, musculoskeletal, range of motion, reliability

INTRODUCTION AND PURPOSE

Lower extremity posture is related to gestational age in newborns (Dubowitz & Dubowitz, 1981). The fullterm newborn demonstrates hip flexion, knee flexion, and dorsiflexion contractures secondary to the prolonged period the fetus spends with the legs folded up against the trunk (Harris, Simmons, Ritchie, Mullett, & Myerbert, 1990). In contrast, a predominance of extensor posture in the lower extremities of preterm infants has been noted by several researchers (Dubowitz, Dubowitz, & Goldberg, 1970; Harris et al., 1990; Heriza, 1982). The preterm infant demonstrates less flexion as a result of being born prior to the completion of rapid growth that occurs during the last trimester of pregnancy.

Muscle and tendon length can be affected by prolonged positioning of the infant's limbs. Range of motion has been assessed in both fullterm and preterm infants (Harris et al., 1990); however, traditional range of motion measurements only account for the maximum stretch of the muscle belly and tendon as a unit. Confinement of the infant in utero could theoretically lead to changes in the tendon, muscle belly, or both.

Understanding what has changed and how this may affect the ability of the muscle to activate around the joint may provide insight into movement changes observed during development of the infant born preterm.

Determining the influence of muscle and tendon length on active muscle force production may have implications for understanding preterm motor development and decisions regarding the need for early intervention. The length-tension curve provides a framework to understand the potential effect of change in tendon or muscle belly on movement (Latash, 1998). The length tension curve illustrates that muscle force production is affected by the length or relationship of the muscle belly fibers. In other words, the amount of force produced by a muscle depends on the amount of stretch in the muscle belly itself or the amount of overlap of the actin and myosin filaments within the muscle. More overlap of the actin and myosin filaments results in the ability to produce greater force in the muscle. As a result, changing the overlap of the muscle fibers will alter where in the range around the joint the muscle can produce force, however, the total range the muscle could produce force would not change. Lengthening the muscle belly, or increasing the number of sacromeres, would likely lead to an increase in the actual joint range the muscle could produce force or activate around the joint.

Additionally, the length of the tendon can change how much stretch is exerted on the muscle. Lengthening the tendon would change the overlap of the muscle fibers by decreasing the stretch on them. Shortening the tendon would cause stretch in the muscle to occur earlier in the range. Alterations to the muscle belly or the tendon could lead to changes in functional movement by altering where in the range force can be produced.

Differences in motor development of preterm and fullterm infants have been reported that may be related to the muscle/tendon unit length. Heriza (1982) examined infant kicking in fullterm and preterm infants. She reported a more extended position of the ankle during kicking and a larger excursion in active ankle movement of preterm infants. These changes could be explained by differences in the muscle/tendon unit length. Differences in preterm infant ankle movement during kicking could be explained by a lengthened gastrocnemius/soleus muscle and/or tendon. Thus, increased length in the gastrocnemius/soleus tendon could result in muscle contractions occurring in a more extended position.

Cioni et al. (1993) reported that when compared with fullterm infants, preterm infants frequently demonstrated a higher frequency of toe-touch contact when beginning to walk and that preterm infants observed using toe-touch contact, demonstrated an extensor dominance during supine kicking and extension at 6 weeks of age. In contrast, fullterm infants more frequently demonstrated a foot flat position when beginning to walk. This finding may be the result of differences in muscle and/or tendon length. Specifically, a change in the length of the gastrocnemius/soleus muscle/tendon unit could explain activation of the gastrocnemius/soleus muscle around the ankle joint during a more extended position in preterm infants during early walking. Analysis of videotapes taken at 6 weeks of age, indicated that infants who used toe-touch contact when beginning to walk demonstrated extensor dominance during supine kicking and extension in the legs during ventral and axillary suspension compared with infants who used flat-foot contact (chi-squared 5.97, df = 1, p < 0.02). Cioni et al. (1993) suggest that differences in walking were not explained by neurological examination findings, although data analysis was not performed. The perspective that ankle movement is not related to positive neurological findings suggests that research is needed to examine whether there are differences in development of the musculoskeletal system of preterm and fullterm infants.

The quality of walking observed in children born preterm by Samsom, de Groot, Cranendonk, Bzemer, Lafeber, and Fetters (2002) may be a reflection of the musculoskeletal system. These authors examined 63 children born preterm at 7 years for a variety of abilities including quality of walking. The children demonstrated, among other problems, difficulty walking on their heels (41%) and were incapable of walking on their toes (27%). These problems could be the result of changes in the ability to move into dorsiflexion (lengthen the gastrocnemius/soleus) or activate the gastrocnemius/soleus in the range needed at the ankle.

A better understanding of the relationship between muscle and tendon extensibility and active movements of the legs has implications for physical and occupational therapy practice. Conventional methods for measuring passive and active range of motion do not differentiate where in the range the muscle belly is lengthening and where the tendon is fully lengthened. A reliable and feasible way to measure changes in the muscle belly and the tendon would enable therapists to examine if changes in the muscle/tendon unit are related to changes in joint movement observed during function, specifically supine kicking and the development of walking.

Tardieu et al. (1982) developed a clinical method of distinguishing muscle and tendon extensibility of the gastrocnemius/soleus muscle that may be applicable to examine muscle extensibility in newborn infants. These authors suggest that muscle extensibility is important for understanding active range of movement. The procedure was examined for the gastrocnemius/soleus muscle, as the authors state this muscle is important for walking, which is frequently the focus of treatment in children diagnosed with cerebral palsy. A_O is defined as the point in tibiocalcaneal range where the slack is taken up in the Achille's tendon and the muscle belly was shortened. Clinically, this point in the range is measured by palpating the Achille's tendon and measuring the angle when palpation of the tendon revealed minimal stiffening. A_{Max} is defined as the point in the tibiocalcaneal range where the tendon and the muscle belly were fully lengthened. Clinically, this point in the range is measured at maximum dorsiflexion of the tibiocalcaneal joint. The difference between these two measures is labeled A_O to A_{Max}. A_O to A_{Max} reflects the passive extensibility of the gastrocnemius/soleus muscle.

Reliability of this clinical measure of muscle extensibility of the gastrocnemius/soleus was estimated when compared to actual torque measures taken at the ankle. Tardieu et al. (1982) reported results using minimal torque and maximal torque that were very similar to the measurements taken using the clinical method. While this method could be useful in investigating gastrocnemius/soleus muscle and tendon length difference in the preterm and fullterm populations, reliability has not been examined.

The purpose of this study was to investigate the inter-rater and test-retest reliability for measuring muscle extensibility of the gastrocnemius/soleus muscle in preterm and fullterm newborn infants using the method developed by Tardieu et al. (1982). This method of measuring muscle extensibility relies on using a goniometer to measure ankle range in a position of maximum dorsiflexion and at a point in the range where palpation reveals minimum tension in the Achille's tendon. Since reliability with older children has been estimated (Tardieu et al., 1982), we hypothesized that this method of measuring muscle extensibility is reliable in newborn infants.

Intraclass correlation coefficients (ICC's) are commonly used to determine the reliability of measurements (Portney & Watkins, 2000). ICC's reflect both the degree of correlation in the measures and the amount of agreement in the ratings (Portney & Watkins, 2000). ICC model 2 and 3 can be used to estimate inter-rater and test-retest reliability. The criterion for good inter-rater and test-retest reliability suggested by Portney and Watkins (2000) (ICC values of .75 or greater) was used in this study.

METHOD

Subjects

Subjects included 41 newborn infants, 21 who were born fullterm and 20 who were born preterm. Subjects were recruited from a local hospital newborn nursery and neonatal intensive care unit (NICU). Medical charts were reviewed to identify infants who met the criteria for fullterm or preterm subjects. All fullterm subjects were born following 38 to 42 weeks gestation, had no known complications during pregnancy or delivery, had an APGAR of 7 or above at 5 minutes, and a normal newborn exam. Preterm subjects were born following 26 to 36 weeks gestation. All preterm subjects had no indications of musculoskeletal impairment, neurological impairment, or genetic abnormalities and were able to tolerate the handling required to take the muscle extensibility measures.

Fullterm infants were enrolled in the study within 48 hours following birth in an attempt to document the gastrocnemius/soleus muscle extensibility at birth. Preterm infants were enrolled in the study prior to term age as soon as the nursing staff or neonatologist reported they had become medically stable. Infants born preterm were measured an average of 15.5 days post birth with a range of 1 to 48 days. The study was approved by the Internal Review Board at the University of Scranton and the Executive Committee at Scranton Community Medical Center. Parents signed an informed consent following explanation of the project.

Instrumentation and Measure

Range of motion at the ankle of each infant was measured with a small 6 inch, 360 degree, clear plastic, goniometer as recommended by Harris, Simons, Ritchie, Mullett, and Myerberg (1990). Two measurements were taken at each infant's ankle, A_O and A_{Max}. A_O was defined as the point in the ankle range of motion where minimal tension was palpated in the Achille's tendon (Tardieu et al., 1982). This measure was assumed to reflect a position of no muscle belly stretch. A_{Max} was defined as the position of full stretch into ankle dorsiflexion and reflects a position of maximum muscle belly stretch (Tardieu et al., 1982).

Procedure

Two physical therapists performed the measurements. Examiner 1 (MGB) is trained in Als' Neonatal Individual Developmental Care and

Assessment Program (Als, 1984), and is experienced measuring muscle extensibility in newborn infants. Examiner 2 (PL) is an experienced physical therapist, who prior to the study, had not measured range of motion in newborn infants. Examiner 2 practiced the technique prior to data collection and then data collection was initiated in the newborn nursery. Data collection for this reliability assessment was initiated with ten infants born fullterm. After collecting data on ten infants born fullterm in the newborn nursery, examinations on infants born preterm were initiated. Initially, the second examiner reported difficulty handling the small limbs of the newborns and the goniometer simultaneously; however, following collection on the first few newborns this examiner felt more comfortable and found measuring the infants easier.

Prior to data collection, examiner 2 was educated on the physiological instability and states demonstrated by infants born preterm. All monitoring of the infants born fullterm and the infants born preterm was carried out by examiner 1. At no time was examiner 2 left alone to monitor the infant's state or physiological stability. In all cases, a nurse was present during data collection for questions or concerns.

All fullterm infants were measured prior to 48 hours of age. All of the preterm infants were measured prior to term age. Seven of the preterm infants (35%) were measured prior to 48 hours of age and ten (50%) were measured within a week of birth. No subjects were eliminated secondary to inability to maintain a state 1, 2, or 4. Twenty-eight infants (68.3%) remained in state 1, 2, or 4 throughout measurement. Five infants (12.2%) moved into a brief state 3 (drowsy). Five infants (12.2%) moved into a brief state 5 (active, awake). Three infants (7.3%) moved between a state 5 to state 3 for a brief period; two of these infants were in a state 5 when the examiner began measurement. The examiner easily assisted these three infants into a state 2. No infants were ever observed in a state 6 (crying).

The examiners attempted to measure each infant midway between feedings unless nursing requested another time. A nurse was consulted about each infant's feeding schedule and any medical tests that might interfere with scheduling. Parents and nursing approved when measurement occurred with one or both parents frequently present during measurement.

Measurements were made when the infants were asleep or in a quiet, alert state as defined by Als (1984) and Brazelton (1984) (state 1, 2, or 4). During testing, if an infant was not in a state 1, 2, or 4, the examiners ceased measurement and only re-initiated measurement when the infant returned to state 1, 2, or 4. Infants were placed in either a sidelying or supine position with all measurements occurring in the same position. For preterm subjects in the NICU, oxygen saturation, respiration, color, and behavior were constantly monitored to ensure each infant was physiologically stable. The leg that was least restrained by monitoring devices or ankle identification tags was selected for testing. Socks and blankets were removed from the selected lower extremity. Every effort was made to keep the infant, minus the leg being measured, swaddled and warm. Both the infants born fullterm and preterm tolerated the handling required to take the measurements. Careful monitoring of the preterm infants proved helpful. If the infant's oxygen saturation decreased, respiratory rate became irregular, or color degraded, measurement was ceased for a brief period to allow re-stabilization of the infant's vitals. In all instances, this was sufficient and measurement could be reinitiated. No subject was removed from the study secondary to poor tolerance of the measurement procedure.

Each physical therapist measured A_O and A_{Max} twice. Examiners measured in a random order. A small goniometer was placed on the lateral side of the selected leg while the hip and knee were maintained in a position of maximum extension. Each therapist palpated the Achille's tendon while measuring A_O, to determine where in the range minimum tension occurred in the Achille's tendon (Figure 1). The infant's foot was moved into full dorsiflexion and A_{max} was measured (Figure 2). Measurements were recorded on separate pieces of paper initially to blind each examiner to the measurements of the other. The measurements took approximately 5 to 10 minutes to complete. Measurement times were slightly longer for the preterm infants secondary to increased care in handling and preparation for measurement.

The angles corresponding to A_O and A_{Max} were recorded on a data sheet following each measure. Dorsiflexion was recorded as a positive degree and plantarflexion was recorded as a negative degree with neutral ankle position referred to as zero degrees. Following measurement, infants were redressed and placed in the position they were found prior to measurement.

Data Analysis

Range of motion measurements were entered onto a spreadsheet and Statistical Package for Social Sciences (SPSS) version 9.0 was used to calculate the ICC's and confidence intervals. Data was entered onto spreadsheets for fullterm and preterm subjects. Confidence levels determined the range of values that contains each ICC at 95% level of confi-

FIGURE 1. Measurement of A_o on an infant born fullterm.

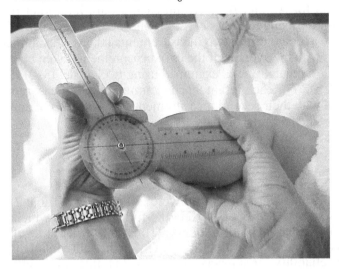

FIGURE 2. Measurement of A_{max} on an infant born fullterm.

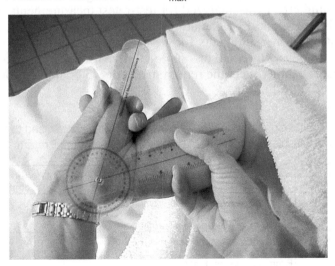

dence. Reliability was examined separately for fullterm and preterm infants and for A_O and A_{Max} within each group. Inter-rater reliability was examined using ICC model (2, 2) (Shrout & Fleiss, 1979). For each infant, the average of the two measurements taken by examiner 1 was compared with the average of the two measurements taken by examiner 2. Test-retest reliability was examined using ICC model (3, 2) (Shrout & Fleiss, 1979). For each infant, each examiner's first measurement was compared with their second measurement. The methods of analysis for inter-rater and test-retest reliability are listed in Table 1.

RESULTS

ICC's for inter-rater reliability were .90 or higher (Table 2), except for inter-rater reliability of A_{Max} in the fullterm infants which was .86 (95% Confidence Interval of .66 to .94). Examiner learning effect was examined for inter-rater reliability of A_{Max} in the fullterm infants by calculating reliability for subjects 11-21 (n = 11). Inter-rater reliability of A_{Max} for subjects 11 to 21 was .93 (95% Confidence Interval of .69 to .98). All ICC's calculated for inter-rater reliability meet the requirements of .75 or above (Portney & Watkins, 2000).

ICC's for test-retest reliability were .90 or higher (Table 3). Examiner learning effect was analyzed for test-retest measurements of A_{Max} in the fullterm infants by calculating reliability for subjects 11 to 21 (n = 11). Test-retest measurements for A_{Max} for subjects 11 to 21 was .94 (95% Confidence Interval of .86 to .98). All ICC's calculated for test-retest reliability meet the requirements of .75 or above (Portney & Watkins, 2000).

TABLE 1. Calculations of Intraclass Correlation Coefficients Used to Examine Reliability of Muscle Extensibility Measures in Fullterm and Preterm Infants

Reliability Assessed	Comparisons	Measurements Compared
Inter-Rater Model (2,2)	Examiner 1–Average measurements Compared to Examiner 2–Average measurements	A_O, A_{Max}
Test-retest Model (3,2)	Examiner's first measurements Compared to Examiner's second measurements	A_O, A_{Max}

A_O = shortened muscle belly and tendon; A_{Max} = lengthened muscle belly and tendon

DISCUSSION

The high ICC's support the hypothesis that the method of measuring muscle extensibility in the gastrocnemius/soleus proposed by Tardieu et al. (1982) is reliable in fulterm and preterm newborn infants. The only ICC lower than .90 was the inter-rater reliability in the fulterm infants on A_{Max}. However, for the last 11 subjects born fulterm, the ICC (2, 1) for inter-rater reliability was .93. This increase in inter-rater reli-

TABLE 2. Intraclass Correlation Coefficient Values and 95% Confidence Interval for Inter-Rater Reliability

Inter-Rater Comparison	ICC (2,2)	95% Confidence Interval
1st and 2nd fulterm A_O measurements for examiner 1 compared to the 1st and 2nd fulterm A_O measurement for examiner 2 (n = 21)	.97	.90 - .99
1st and 2nd preterm A_O measurement for examiner 1 compared to the 1st and 2nd preterm A_O measurement for examiner 2 (n = 20)	.96	.91 - .99
1st and 2nd fulterm measurement of A_{Max} for examiner 1 compared to the 1st and 2nd fulterm A_{Max} measurement for examiner 2 (n = 21) ** eliminating 1st ten subjects (n = 11)	.86 .93**	.66 - .94 .69 - .98**
1st and 2nd preterm measurement of A_{Max} for examiner 1 compared to the 1st and 2nd preterm A_{Max} measurement for examiner 2 (n = 20)	.95	.89 - .98

TABLE 3. Intraclass Correlation Coefficient Values and 95% Confidence Intervals for Test-Retest Reliability

Test-Retest Comparison	ICC (3,2)	95% Confidence Interval
1st fulterm A_O measurement for examiner 1 and 2 compared to the 2nd fulterm A_O measurement for examiner 1 and 2 (n = 21)	.97	.96 - .99
1st preterm A_O measurement for examiner 1 and 2 compared to the 2nd preterm A_O measurement for examiner 1 and 2 (n = 20)	.98	.96 - .99
1st fulterm A_{Max} measurement for examiner 1 and 2 compared to the 2nd fulterm A_{Max} measurements for examiner 1 and 2 (n = 21) ** eliminating 1st ten subjects (n = 11)	.91 .94**	.83 - .95 .86 - .98**
1st preterm A_{Max} measurement for examiner 1 and 2 compared to the 2nd preterm A_{Max} measurements for examiner 1 and 2 (n = 20)	.97	.94 - .98

ability suggests that reliability increased with practice. Subjects born fullterm were the majority of the initial subjects measured, because they were easier to recruit than the subjects born preterm. These first 10 subjects were the second examiners initial attempts at measuring muscle extensibility in infants. The lower intraclass correlation for the first 10 fullterm subjects appears to reflect the fact examiner 2 was learning how much pressure to exert on a newborn's ankle during measurement of A_{Max}.

An additional reason inter-rater reliability may have increased following the first ten fullterm subjects is that testing A_{Max} was refined during this study. During routine inspection of measurements following data collection, the examiners noted that the A_{Max} score increased on each subsequent measurement. The authors hypothesized that the gastrocnemius/soleus was stretched by the initial one or two measures of A_{Max} and with subsequent measure of A_{Max} the muscle length increased. Approximately one quarter of the way through data collection, the examiners decided to stretch the gastrocnemius/soleus muscle two or three times prior to measuring A_{Max}. This change in stretching the muscle belly prior to measurement affected the infants born fullterm to a greater degree than the infants born preterm since data were collected on the subjects born fullterm were gathered prior to the subjects born preterm. This is supported by the fact that the test-retest reliability for the infants born fullterm A_{Max} measurement was lower than for the infants born preterm and the test-retest reliability increased for fullterm subjects 11 to 21.

This method of measuring muscle extensibility is feasible to use with fullterm and preterm newborns. The fact that measurement was tolerated so well by all of the subjects suggests that this measurement can be used with the often-fragile preterm infant. Careful monitoring of preterm infants should be done by a therapist experienced in working with fragile newborns. The infant should be closely monitored during measurement of muscle extensibility to ensure oxygen saturation, heart rate, respiration, and color are stable.

Reliability for measuring muscle extensibility of the gastrocnemius/soleus muscle can be achieved in the clinical setting. The fact that there was no special training for examiner 2, suggests that a therapist with general skills in measuring range of motion can achieve reliability with this goniometric measure and minimal practice. This does not mean someone without experience in the Neonatal Intensive Care Unit should provide services in the Neonatal Intensive Care Unit (Sweeney, Heriza, Reilly, Smith, & VanSant, 1999). Rather, the results indicate that extensive training is not necessary to achieve reliability for the measurement of muscle extensibility. We recommend that a therapist practice on ten or more newborns prior to documentation of muscle extensibility as part of clinical practice. It is also suggested that the ankle be moved through the full range of motion including a brief stretch of the muscle belly in the lengthened position prior to actual measurement of A_{Max}.

In addition to the feasibility and reliability of this method, measuring muscle extensibility can be done quickly. Measuring both A_O and A_{Max} twice takes approximately five to ten minutes. If this measurement adds valuable information to an assessment, it has the added benefit of taking a very short amount of time to perform and requires only a small goniometer and minimal training.

With evidence that measurement of muscle extensibility is reliable and feasible, further research is needed to examine whether muscle extensibility affects differences reported in infant kicking reported by Heriza (1982) or the differences seen in early foot contact reported by Cioni et al. (1993). Further research is needed to determine if muscle extensibility differs between infants born fullterm and preterm. If differences in muscle extensibility do exist, determination of how muscle extensibility affects movement during function, such as kicking and walking, should be examined. Evidence of a cause-effect relationship is needed prior to recommending interventions to alter muscle extensibility in infants born preterm.

REFERENCES

Als, H. (1984). *Neonatal Individualized Developmental Care and Assessment Program (NIDCAP)*. Boston, MA: Children's Hospital.

Brazelton, T.B. (1984). *Neonatal Behavioral Assessment Scale, 2nd Edition. Clinics in Developmental Medicine, No. 88*. Philadelphia, PA: JB Lippencott.

Cioni, G., Duchini, F., Milianti, B., Paolicelli, P.B., Sicola, E., Boldrini, A., & Ferrari, A. (1993). Differences and variations in the patterns of early independent walking. *Early Human Development*, 35, 193-205.

Dubowitz, L.M.S. & Dubowitz, V. (1981). The neurological assessment of the preterm and full-term newborn infant. *Clinics in Developmental Medicine*, 79, 1-103.

Dubowitz, L.M.S., Dubowitz, V., & Goldberg, C. (1970). Clinical assessment of gestational age in the newborn infant. *Journal of Pediatrics*, 77(1), 1-10.

Harris, M.B., Simons, C.J.R., Ritchie, S.K., Mullett, M.D., & Myerberg, D.Z. (1990). Joint range of motion development in premature infants. *Physical Therapy*, 2, 185-191.

Heriza, C.B. (1982). Organization of Leg Movements in Preterm Infants. *Physical Therapy*, 68(9), 1340-1346.

Latash, M.L. (1998). Neurophysiological Basis of Movement. Champaign, IL: Human Kinetics.

Portney, L.G. & Watkins, M.P. (2000). *Foundations of Clinical Research: Applications to Practice, 2nd ed.* Upper Saddle River, NJ: Prentice Hall.

Samsom, J.F., de Groot, L., Cranendonk, A., Bezemer, P.D., Lafeber, H.N., & Fetter, W.P.F. (2002). *Journal of Child Neurology*, 17, 325-332.

Shrout, P.E. & Fleiss, J.L. (1979). Intraclass correlations: Uses in assessing rater reliability. *Psychological Bulletin*, 86(2), 420-428.

Sweeney, J.K., Heriza, C.B., Reilly, M.A., Smith, C., & VanSant, A.F. (1999). Practice guidelines for the physical therapist in the neonatal intensive care unit (NICU). *Pediatric Physical Therapy*, 11(3), 119-132.

Tardieu, C., de la Tour, H., Bret, M.D., & Tardieu, G. (1982). Muscle hypoextensibility in children with cerebral palsy: I. Clinical and experimental observations. *Archives of Physical Medicine and Rehabilitation*, 63, 97-102.

Index

Numbers followed by "n" indicate notes.

T - #0549 - 101024 - C0 - 212/152/11 - PB - 9780789025616 - Gloss Lamination